A Healthcare Students Introduction to Global Health

Alison Fiander • Grace Fry
Editors

A Healthcare Students Introduction to Global Health

Low- and Middle Income Countries

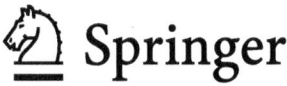 Springer

Editors
Alison Fiander
Emeritus Chair Obstetrics and Gynaecology
School of Medicine, Cardiff University
Cardiff, UK

Grace Fry
School of Medicine
Cardiff University
Cardiff, UK

ISBN 978-3-031-66562-2   ISBN 978-3-031-66563-9   (eBook)
https://doi.org/10.1007/978-3-031-66563-9

This Springer imprint is published by the registered company Springer Nature Switzerland AG
The registered company address is: Gewerbestrasse 11, 6330 Cham, Switzerland

If disposing of this product, please recycle the paper.

Preface

The Importance of Global Health and how this Book Came to Be!

In today's interconnected world, the realm of global health is becoming increasingly relevant. There are numerous reasons why Global Health should be an essential component of undergraduate healthcare curricula, yet curiously, global health is seldom a formal component of undergraduate healthcare curricula.

Integrating global health into undergraduate healthcare curricula allows students to develop a broader perspective and enables them to understand healthcare challenges in different parts of the world, analysing how global factors impact the healthcare systems in their own country, including the climate emergency and the part healthcare contributes to greenhouse emissions.

Global health education highlights the shared nature of health conditions across the globe. It empowers students to identify and tackle health issues that transcend national boundaries, such as the evolving demographics of infectious and non-communicable diseases, as well as the emergence of global health crises. Students studying global health gain cultural competence, which enables them to work effectively with diverse populations, both at home and abroad. This cultivates the ability to provide culturally sensitive care and formulate apt healthcare strategies in multicultural settings.

A study of global health exposes students to diverse cultural, socioeconomic, and ethical perspectives and helps students understand social determinants of health. This enables healthcare professionals to address health inequities both locally and globally, becoming advocates for change and the reduction of health disparities.

In an interconnected world, global health emergencies can surface suddenly, as exemplified by the Covid-19 pandemic. By integrating global health into the curriculum, healthcare students gain the knowledge and skills necessary to respond adeptly to crises such as epidemics, natural disasters, and refugee health emergencies.

Healthcare professionals are increasingly involved in global health diplomacy and global health teaching equips students with the necessary understanding of global health governance, policies, and diplomacy, enabling them to contribute to national and international health initiatives. This, in turn, opens a wealth of employment opportunities across diverse professional settings, encompassing international organizations, non-governmental entities, and public health institutions.

Considering this, one of the editors, Alison Fiander, developed a week-long 'Short course in Global Health' for second year medical undergraduates, as a Student Selected Component (SSC) for the Medical School at Cardiff University. As part of the week students researched, wrote about, and presented different aspects of Global Health, which subsequently formed the basis and chapters of this book. The Global Health SSC is now being led by one of the other authors contributing to the book.

Grace Fry, the second editor, undertook to edit some of the 'chapters' as a third year SSC at Cardiff Medical School (although this turned out to take much longer than the time specified for an SSC!).

Aimed at healthcare students, i.e. medical, nursing, and allied professionals, this textbook covers a broad range of topics in Global Health in short accessible chapters. We hope that it is useful for your studies and that it may perhaps encourage you to explore a career in Global Health.

Cardiff, UK   Alison Fiander
                                                                                                    Grace Fry

Contents

About the Editors

Alison Fiander was appointed Chair of Obstetrics and Gynaecology at Cardiff University in 2002. Having worked in Sub-Saharan Africa for 4 years earlier in her career, Alison has a passionate commitment to mitigating global maternal mortality and morbidity. In 2015, Alison left Cardiff University to serve as the Clinical Lead for the Royal College of Obstetricians and Gynaecologists (RCOG) Leading Safe Choices programme, imparting sexual reproductive health training to healthcare professionals in Tanzania and South Africa. She subsequently became the Clinical Lead for the RCOG Centre for Global Women's Health overseeing the development of the RCOG Essential Gynaecology Skills course (now renamed Gynaecological Health Matters) for Low- and Middle-Income countries (LMIC).

Alison retired from the RCOG in 2018 but continues work as an independent consultant in Global Women's Health in addition to teaching global health to both undergraduates and postgraduates and directing an online postgraduate diploma/ MSc in International Women's Health.

Grace Fry has now graduated from the School of Medicine at Cardiff University. She has a longstanding interest in Global Health, especially the health of refugee and asylum seekers. She is keen that these topics gain greater prominence in the undergraduate curriculum.

As a member of 'Students for Global Health' society committee, she co-organised a Cardiff University conference titled 'Refugees: Welcome Here' in 2022. She is also a keen linguist and traveller, undertaking her Women, Child, and Family medical placement in Nantes, France. Having graduated, she plans to complete a Global Health/Women's Health MSc with the intention of working in this field in the future.

Chapter 1
What Is Global Health?

Jacqueline Boulton

1.1 What Is Global Health?

At first glance, the answer to this question may seem quite straightforward; indeed, during the author's extensive experience of teaching global health modules to BSc and MSc level healthcare students, this is often the starting assumption. This is also borne out of experience in supervising the dissertations of students who initially state that they want to focus on global health but struggle to identify a specific aspect and question to explore.

Before going any further then, let's start by considering how global health is best defined. Again, this may not be quite as easy as it had perhaps appeared. One way of ensuring a comprehensive and succinct definition is to first spend time considering what global health incorporates. Perhaps at this point, you would like to briefly pause and come up with your own definition.

Underlying any definition is a central tenant that health is a human right and therefore achieving global health 'for all' is a recognised and agreed upon aim [1]. This was of course embedded in the constitution of the World Health Organisation (WHO) from its inception in 1946 [2], but achieving such a laudable goal seems to be ever more complex as will become apparent throughout the different chapters of this book.

When undertaking academic writing, healthcare students can understandably become overwhelmed by finding appropriate sources of support. Within the global health paradigm, the issue is more likely to centre around becoming overwhelmed by the plethora of information available. It is essential to ensure robust and up-to date data are accessed and that that data is used appropriately to make relevant cross comparison. Another frequently asked question centres around how 'old' references

J. Boulton (✉)
King's College, London, UK
e-mail: Jacqui.boulton@kcl.ac.uk

© The Author(s), under exclusive license to Springer Nature
Switzerland AG 2024
A. Fiander, G. Fry (eds.), *A Healthcare Students Introduction to Global Health*,
https://doi.org/10.1007/978-3-031-66563-9_1

can be. Whilst statistical data relating to Global Health needs to be the most up to date available, there is also scope for seminal referencing particularly when considering how Global Health is defined. In terms of defining the concept of global health, the seminal definition by Koplan et al. in 2009 still appears to be the most widely accepted. Koplan defines global health as 'an area for study, research, and practice that places a priority on improving health and achieving health equity for all people worldwide' [3]. But how on earth can this be achieved?

1.2   Establishing a Global Health Paradigm

The term 'global health' itself is a relatively new 'label'. Its scope and associated concepts have evolved throughout centuries reflecting changes in biological understanding, socioeconomic and political contexts alongside contemporary threats to health [4]. A whistle stop tour providing brief insight into the key historical landmarks and emphasis will help healthcare students to understand how the current collaborative and interconnected nature of the discipline has evolved [5].

1.2.1   Historical Perspectives

In a similar way that psychology has grappled with the nature vs. nurture debate for centuries [6], there has been an historical rivalry between theories of disease causation. This rivalry gathered momentum in the latter part of the nineteenth century under the catalyst of the industrial revolution. This period heralded several key inventions and discoveries relating to both biological causation of disease (germ theory) and environmental causation (miasma theory) [4, 7].

1.2.2   Public Health

In the UK, increasing awareness of the links between human health and environmental factors, specifically sanitation, was expedited by the work of John Snow and others following a series of cholera, typhoid and influenza pandemics. In 1848, this led to the establishment of the general board of health, a body charged with the centralised administrative and regulation of Public Health [4]. Its scope and emphasis were enshrined within the first UK public health act [8].

1.2.3 Tropical Medicine

During this period, a second wave of colonial expansion was also taking place bringing with it an ongoing threat posed by both new and re-emerging Infectious diseases. A number of key scientific inventions and discoveries relating to biological disease causation came to the fore hugely helped by further advances in microscopy following on from the invention of the first microscope in 1590 [9]. This included the identification and categorisation of some significant pathogens found in the mosquito-infested tropical regions of colonial discovery [10, 11]. It also saw the fruition of work by several scientists to find a way of eradicating smallpox. The successful creation of a smallpox vaccine was ultimately credited to Jenner who became hailed as 'the father of immunology' [12].

1.2.4 International Health

'International health' was already a term of considerable currency in the late nineteenth and early twentieth centuries when it referred primarily to the increasing need to focus upon attempts to prevent the spread of epidemics across international boundaries.

Awareness that 'no man is an island' became official in the early 1900s as similar bodies to the UK board of Health began to collaborate across Europe. In Paris, the Office Internationale d'Hygiène Publique was formed. Through its auspices, an international set of rules was developed around the quarantining of ships to prevent the spread of plague and cholera [4]. Later, and shortly after the ending of the First World War, the League of Nations Health Organisation was established in Geneva [13]. Under its governance, several international commissions were set up to combat the threat of specific diseases. This institution was a precursor to the establishment of the United Nations (UN) in 1945 and its health-related arm, the WHO.

As the century progressed, further developments both about the way in which diseases are spread and the relationship of environmental factors upon this continued to emerge. This led to a more advanced theoretical understanding of the need to incorporate, expand upon and synthesise approaches. The Declaration of Primary Health Care and the goal of 'Health for All in the Year 2000' advocated an 'intersectoral' and multidimensional approach to health and socioeconomic development with an emphasis on 'appropriate technology' [14]. It also urged active community participation in healthcare and health education at every level. The working out of these principles and the differing extent to which the components were emphasised however remained a source of debate. In 1993, the World Bank, which had become increasingly influential, published the World Development Report: Investing in Health [15]. This became very significant for the future of health priorities in the global arena and gave rise to a more collaborative approach incorporating multiple non-governmental organisations (NGOs), private donors, internationally influential foundations and multilateral agencies. Quick-fix solutions such as short-term selective programmes were frequently prioritised over the longer term aims of improving health through an emphasis on the growth of primary healthcare. Alliances were formed with a focus on a specific target, e.g., Roll Back Malaria, 1998 [16] and the Global Alliance for Vaccines and Immunisation [17]. These global health partnerships multiplied quickly reaching 70 within a few years [18].

1.2.5   Global Health: From MDGs to SDGs [19]

Against this background, there was a major review of management, strategy and priorities of the WHO. There was also great concern and mistrust of international economic institutions and a need for a complete review within the UN itself. As the twentieth century ended, several key UN summits took place, ultimately culminating in the signing of the United Nations Millennium Declaration, in September 2000. This declaration was signed by 189 countries, and its aims were enshrined within the UN Millennium Development Goals (MDGs). Within the health realm, these eight goals sought to combine the historical rivalry between biological and environmental causations and solutions of illness. Specific goals were set which were measurable according to specific targets and indicators. Three of the eight were specifically focused on health with the remaining five very much interlinked by a broader focus on social development [19, 20]. During this period, the term International Health was replaced by Global Health.

Much progress was made during the 15 years that the MDGs covered, but in 2015, these were replaced by the Sustainable Development Goals (SDGs). The SDGs seek to broaden areas for action with greater specificity. They also acknowledged that all countries across the globe have a vital role to play, albeit that the effort and resources needed to meet each specific goal will vary considerably, though hopefully more equitably [5]. There are 17 goals, 169 targets and 231 indices through which progress can be measured. Goal 3 focuses specifically on Health. However, there are other specific indicators related to health embedded within other goals, and each target has some connection to the overall state of the world's health. Progress for each goal, target and indicator can be seen using the SDG dashboard through which data for making cross comparison by country and year can also be generated [21].

1.3   The Language of Global Health (Fig. 1.1)

Like most disciplines, Global health has some key terms and concepts that must be understood by any healthcare student who wishes to study research or practice within its arena [3]. It is essential to understand this; only then can any meaningful

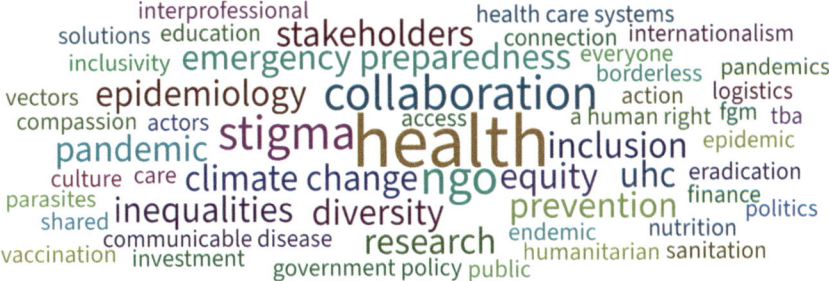

Fig. 1.1 Infographic word cloud depicting key concepts, terms and considerations underpinning Global Health

cross comparison of health between countries be made. Moreover, such measurement is essential in arguing for and allocating funding. It is also paramount to consider the way in which countries and continents are described globally [22].

This 'language of Global Health' has also evolved over time. An understanding of current terms such as 'stakeholders' and 'capacity building' together with key concepts such as 'Capacity Building, Universal Health Coverage (UHC) and Disability Adjusted Life Years (DALYs)' is essential. The Centres for Disease Control and Prevention (CDC) has produced a helpful section on this [23].

In terms of the language of Global health, healthcare students will find it reassuring to note that 'Everyone who works cross-culturally and cross-linguistically will make mistakes' [24]. The first key conundrum is how to refer to countries and regions when seeking to make cross comparison.

1.3.1 First World vs. Third World

It is always important to consider the origins of a definition including the background of the individual or the group who have defined it. Moreover, it is crucial that the language used does not reinforce colonial overtones [24]. During the cold war era of the 1950s, for example, the world was divided into three groups. In this definition, 'First world' comprised the United States, Western Europe and its allies. Countries of the communist block were incorporated within the term 'Second world', and the remaining group of countries, many of which were former colonies, were grouped en masse into the Third world. Inherent in this definition is also a hierarchical assumption that first is best.

1.3.2   Developed vs. Developing Countries

Perhaps a more frequently used subdivision is that of 'developing' and 'developed' countries. There seems to be no clear basis for this definition. Furthermore, it begs the question 'developing to what?'; the constitution of the grey area between the two is unclear. Again, there is a clear hierarchical component and an inherent assumption that 'developed countries' constitute some sort of utopia to which lesser countries should aspire in order to be 'complete'.

1.3.3   North vs. South

Another way of categorising the world's countries is the North–South divide. Whilst this may seem clear cut, it has also developed hierarchical associations with countries in the North being assumed to be more prosperous than those in South. A cursory glance at the World Bank definition of countries by income [25] may seem to support this generalisation. However, there are plenty of high-income countries in the South, e.g. Australia and New Zealand, and extremely impoverished countries in the North, e.g. Haiti.

In his excellent book 'Factfulness', Hans Rosling and colleagues demonstrate that the classic assumptions upon which all the above categories are made rely on substantially outdated perceptions [26]. Healthcare students who would prefer to digest this information in a video format are directed to Rosling's earlier TED talk entitled 'The Best Stats You've Ever Seen' [27].

1.4   Can Meaningful Comparison Be Made Between Countries (and If so How)?

A more factual categorization and one that is frequently used is according to income. The most used classification here is that developed by the world bank which groups countries according to income. These categories are based on GNI per capita and are updated every year. There are four groups, low income, low middle income, middle income and high income [25]. Whilst this classification may be a helpful starting point in terms of its clear-cut nature, grouping countries in terms of income alone is of limited value particularly given the importance of the social determinants of health previously discussed. Neither is it the case that an equally proportionate relationship between the income of a country and its healthcare expenditure can be assumed.

In recent times, a whole host of multidimensional indices have evolved to capture a more holistic picture and to incorporate the wider determinants of health and wellbeing [21, 28, 29]. Each of these has a slightly different emphasis in terms of the way in which specific health-related components are envisaged and measured. One of the most frequently used is the Human Development Index Healthcare (HDI) [28]. This is produced annually and gives a specific figure or 'ranking' of all countries who submit data based on three key dimensions and four indices.

The selection of a relevant index is of course highly dependent on the specific aspect of health being considered. It is important that healthcare students weigh up which of the many available indexes is most appropriate to the focus of investigation, being clear about the measure they are using and the reasons for the choice. Nevertheless, it is sometimes interesting to make cross comparison between indexes. This illustrates the differing emphasis that underpins the index itself. For example, in the World Happiness Index, Guatemala ranks 39 out of the 145 countries who submitted data (where 1 is 'highest') [30], but 135 out of 189 countries who submitted data for the HDI (where 1 is 'highest') in the same period [28].

1.4.1 The Impact of COVID

The identification of a new variation of coronavirus (SARS-CoV-2) on 31st December [31] and the subsequent declaration at the end of the following month that this was a Public Health Emergency of International Concern [32] alerted the world to the impending crisis and the resulting disease (subsequently named COVID-19) (Coronavirus Infectious disease 2019). Within 6 weeks, COVID-19 had been declared a pandemic [32]. At the time of writing the WHO reports, 6,948,764 confirmed deaths from the COVID-19 pandemic were reported [33]. The 2022 SDG development report [34] highlights the impact of the crisis on the ability to collect and disseminate meaningful data. This supports widespread acknowledgement that the actual death toll is much greater than reported (see Fig. 1.2). The report also includes infographics for each of the 17 SDG goals which highlight the catastrophic effect on the progress made towards their achievement. In relation to SDG 3.8 for example, despite the laudable aims and efforts of the COVAX alliance, the percentage of people in low-income countries who received at least one dose of vaccine was approximately 17%, compared to around 80% for people in high-income countries [35]. Never has the central promise of the 2030 Agenda for Sustainable Development to 'leave no one behind' [5] been more poignant.

Reported COVID-19 deaths and estimated excess deaths globally, 2020–2021 (millions)

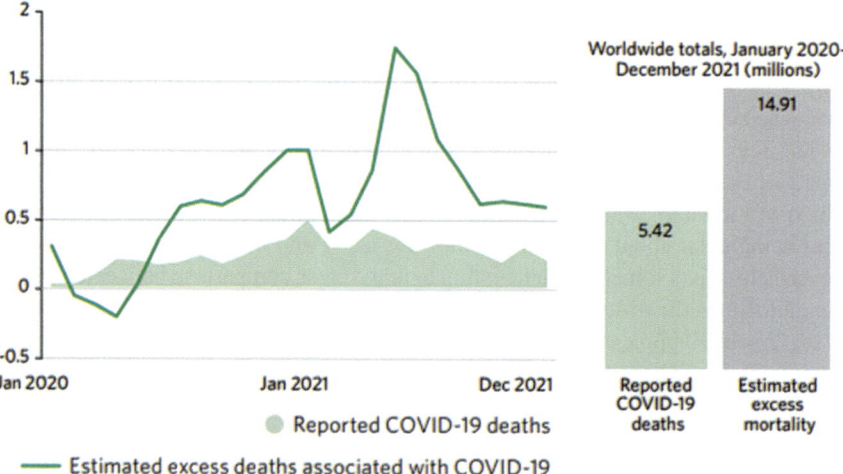

Fig. 1.2 Report on deaths and avoidable deaths from the SDG 2022 [25] report (copyright permission obtained)

References

1. United Nations. Universal Declaration of Human Rights | United Nations [Internet].1945 [cited 2023 June 25] United Nations. Available from: https://www.un.org/en/about-us/universal-declaration-of-human-rights
2. WHO Constitution [Internet]. 1946 [cited 2023 June 25]. Available from: https://www.who.int/about/governance/constitution
3. Koplan JP, Bond TC, Merson MH, Reddy KS, Rodriguez MH, Sewankambo NK, et al. Towards a common definition of global health. Lancet. 2009;373(9679):1993–5.
4. Tulchinsky TH, Varavikova EA. A history of public health. In: Elsevier eBooks [Internet]. 2014. p. 1–42. Available from: https://doi.org/10.1016/b978-0-12-415766-8.00001-x
5. Transforming our world: the 2030 Agenda for Sustainable Development | Department of Economic and Social Affairs [Internet]. 2015 [cited 2023 June 3] Available from: https://sdgs.un.org/2030agenda
6. Witherington DC, Lickliter R. Transcending the nature-nurture debate through epigenetics. Human Devel. 2017;60(2/3):65–8.
7. Holst J. Global health – emergence, hegemonic trends and biomedical reductionism. Global Health. 2020;16(1):42.
8. Alderslade R. The Public Health Act of 1848. BMJ [Internet]. 1998 Aug 29;317(7158):549–550. Available from: https://doi.org/10.1136/bmj.317.7158.549UK government. The Public Health Act 1848.
9. History of microscopes [Internet]. [cited 2023 June 1] Microscope.com. Available from: https://www.microscope.com/education-center/microscopes-101/history-of-microscopes
10. Otsuji Y. History, epidemiology and control of filariasis. Trop Med Health. 2011;39(1 Suppl 2):3–13. https://doi.org/10.2149/tmh.39-1-suppl_2-3. PMID: 22028595; PMCID: PMC3153148.B

11. Cox FE. History of the discovery of the malaria parasites and their vectors. Parasit Vectors. 2010;3(1):5. https://doi.org/10.1186/1756-3305-3-5. PMID: 20205846; PMCID: PMC2825508
12. Riedel S. Edward Jenner and the history of smallpox and vaccination. Proc (Bayl Univ Med Cent). 2005;18(1):21–5. https://doi.org/10.1080/08998280.2005.11928028. PMID: 16200144; PMCID: PMC1200696
13. The Covenant of the League of Nations | UN Geneva [Internet].1902 [cited 2023 June 1] UN GENEVA. Available from: https://www.ungeneva.org/en/about/league-of-nations/covenant
14. Declaration of Alma-Ata, International Conference on Primary Health Care, Alma-Ata, USSR, 6–12 September 1978. http://www.who.int/hpr/NPH/docs/declaration_almaata.pdf
15. World Bank (1993) World Development Report 1993: Investing in Health. https://doi.org/1 0.1596/0-1952-0890-0
16. Yamey G. Roll Back Malaria: a failing global health campaign. BMJ. 2004;328(7448):1086–7. https://doi.org/10.1136/bmj.328.7448.1086. PMID: 15130956; PMCID: PMC406307
17. GAVI, the Vaccine Alliance [Internet]. [cited 2023 June 1] Available from: https://www.gavi.org/
18. Brown TM, Cueto M, Fee E. The World Health Organization and the transition from "international" to "global" public health. Am J Public Health. 2006;96(1):62–72. https://doi.org/10.2105/AJPH.2004.050831. Epub 2005 Dec 1. PMID: 16322464; PMCID: PMC1470434
19. Health in 2015: from MDGs to SDGs [Internet]. 2015. Available from: https://www.who.int/data/gho/publications/mdgs-sdgs
20. United Nations. United Nations Millennium Development goals [Internet]. 2000 [cited 2023 MAY 16] Available from: https://www.un.org/millenniumgoals/
21. Sustainable Development Report 2023 [Internet]. Cited 2023, May 1]. Available from: https://dashboards.sdgindex.org/rankings
22. Khan T, Abimbola S, Kyobutungi C, Pai M. How we classify countries and people-and why it matters. BMJ Glob Health. 2022;7(6):e009704. https://doi.org/10.1136/bmjgh-2022-009704. PMID: 35672117; PMCID: PMC9185389
23. The Centres for Disease Control and Prevention (CDC) Global terminology Considerations [internet]. [Cited 16, May] Available from https://www.cdc.gov/globalhealth/equity/guide/global-term.html
24. The Centres for Disease Control and Prevention (CDC) Cultural Humility and Communication considerations [internet] [Cited 16, May]Available from https://www.cdc.gov/globalhealth/equity/guide/cultural-humility.html
25. World Bank Open Data [Internet]. [Cited 16, May] World Bank Open Data. Available from: https://data.worldbank.org/indicator/NY.GNP.PCAP.CD
26. Rosling H, Rönnlund AR, Rosling O. Factfulness: ten reasons we're wrong about the world–and why things are better than you think. Flatiron Books.
27. Rosling H. The best stats you've ever seen [Internet]. [Cited 2023, May 1] TED Talks. Available from: https://www.ted.com/talks/hans_rosling_the_best_stats_you_ve_ever_seen?language=enRoslin H 2006 'the best stats you've ever seen'
28. HDI Programme UND. Human Development Report 2019: Beyond income, beyond averages, beyond today – inequalities in human development in the 21st Century. United Nations; 2019.
29. About – GHS Index [Internet]. Cited 2023, May 1] GHS Index. 2021. Available from: https://www.ghsindex.org/about/
30. Happiness, Benevolence, and Trust During COVID-19 and Beyond | The World Happiness Report [Internet]. [Cited 2023, May 1] 2022. Available from: https://worldhappiness.report/ed/2022/happiness-benevolence-and-trust-during-covid-19-and-beyond/#ranking-of-happiness-2019-2021
31. Zhou P, Yang XL, Wang XG, Hu B, Zhang L, Zhang W, et al. A pneumonia outbreak associated with a new coronavirus of probable bat origin. Nature. 2020;579(7798):270–3.
32. Coronavirus disease (COVID-19) pandemic [Internet]. 2023. [Cited 2023, May 1] Available from: https://www.who.int/europe/emergencies/situations/covid-19

33. WHO Coronavirus (Covid-19) dashboard [Internet]. WHO Coronavirus (COVID-19) Dashboard with Vaccination Data. [Cited July 5th 2023, July 5th]. Available from: https:// covid19.who.int
34. The Sustainable Development Goals Report 2022 | DISD [Internet]. [Cited 2023, April 26] Available from: https://www.un.org/development/desa/dspd/2022/07/sdgs-report/
35. COVAX [Internet]. 2023 [Cited 2023, May 28]. Available from: https://www.who.int/ initiatives/act-accelerator/covax

Chapter 2
The Global Burden of Disease

Megan Teleri Davies and Ms Eleanor Duckett

2.1 Definitions

Disability-Adjusted Life Years (DALYs) 'One DALY represents the loss of the equivalent of one year of full health. DALYs for a disease or health condition are the sum of the years of life lost to due to premature mortality (YLLs) and the years lived with a disability (YLDs) due to prevalent cases of the disease or health condition in a population'. [2]

Years Lived with a Disability (YLDs) 'One YLD represents the equivalent of one full year of healthy life lost due to disability or ill-health'. [3]

International Classification of Disease (ICD) 'ICD serves a broad range of uses globally and provides critical knowledge on the extent, causes and consequences of human disease and death worldwide via data that is reported and coded with the ICD'. [4]

Socio-Demographic Index (SDI) 'A summary measure that identifies where countries or other geographic areas sit on the spectrum of development. Expressed on a scale of 0–1'. [5]

M. T. Davies (✉)
Llanarth, Ceredigion, UK
e-mail: Megan.Davies25d3e5@wales.nhs.uk

M. E. Duckett
Johnstown, Wrexham, UK
e-mail: elliev@uwclub.net

2.2   Defining Countries Based on Gross National Income (GNI) [6]

Table 2.1

2.3   Socio-Demographic Index (SDI)

The Socio-Demographic Index (SDI) considers a country's:

- Income per capita
- Average years of education
- Fertility rates in females under the age of 25 [7]

The primary factors that influence the globally increasing socio-demographic index include globalisation, urbanisation and development. These have boosted income and wealth by creating more employment and business opportunities. A cascade effect of this has resulted in more people being able to afford education and wealthier lifestyles, including access to alcohol, tobacco and a more diverse diet. Women's rights have increased, encouraging females in higher socio-demographic index countries to work and earn a stable income. This has resulted in fertility rates dropping, again increasing the SDI calculation [8].

2.4   Social Determinants of Health

Social determinants of health (SDH) significantly influence the global burden of disease. There are non-medical factors that can contribute towards health outcomes. They include an individual's occupation, wealth, age, access to healthcare system, lifestyle and geographical location. These shape hey health parameters like life expectancy, morbidity and social norms, while also shaping economic policies and systems. This ultimately impacts the distribution of resources, for example, healthcare access. Health inequities within and between countries are heavily shaped by the Social Determinants of Health. Generally, the lower a country's socio-economic position, the poorer the health of its population [9] (Table 2.2).

Table 2.1 Defining income level		
Low-income country	GNI per capita <$1025
Low middle-income country	GNI per capita $1026–$3995
High middle-income country	GNI per capita $3996–$12,375
High-income country	GNI per capita >$12,376

Table 2.2 Examples of social determinants of health

Financial Status	Employment Expenses Debt Financial support
Environment	Housing Climate Safety Transportation
Education	Accessibility Pre-school education Literacy Higher education Language
Nutrition	Accessibility to food Food hygiene Water and sanitation
Community and Social Care	Neighbourhood Social support Crime Gender, race, ethnicity Cultural norms
Healthcare	Access to health services Pharmaceutical supplies

2.5   Disease Classification

Diseases can be categorised into three categories:

- Communicable, Maternal, Neonatal and Nutritional (CMNN)
- Non-Communicable (NCD)
- Injuries

Communicable, Maternal, Neonatal and Nutritional Diseases Communicable diseases are infectious diseases that can be transmitted between individuals and organisms within the environment, often causing severe symptoms in the host. Maternal and neonatal diseases primarily affect individuals during the antenatal period and childbirth. Nutritional diseases can arise from deficiencies of vitamins and minerals in diets, leading to symptoms and various health consequences [10].

Non-Communicable Diseases A non-infectious disease is a disease that cannot be transmitted directly from one person to another. They are also known as chronic or lifestyle-related diseases [11].

Injuries They include hurt, damage or loss to an individual or to others. This includes a violation of another's rights [12] (Table 2.3).

Table 2.3 Examples of disease categories

Communicable, maternal, neonatal and nutritional diseases (CMNN) examples	Non-communicable diseases (NCDs) examples	Injury examples
HIV/AIDS	Cardiovascular disease—including ischaemic heart disease	Road-traffic accidents
Gastroenteritis and enteric fever (typhoid and paratyphoid)	Cancer	Falls
Tuberculosis	Chronic respiratory disease	Drowning
Malaria and neglected tropical diseases	Diabetes	Natural disasters
Respiratory diseases including MERS-CoV and SARS-Cov2	Neurological disorders—including dementia	Terrorism
Viral haemorrhagic fevers—including Ebola and Lassa fever	Chronic kidney disease	Self-harm
Maternal disorders	Musculoskeletal disorders—including rheumatoid arthritis	Poisoning
Neonatal disorders	Mental disorders—including depression	Fire
Nutritional deficiencies—including iron deficiency and B12 deficiency	Liver diseases	Heat and chemical substances

[10–12]

2.6 Global Deaths

In 2019, most deaths globally were attributed to non-communicable diseases, notably ischaemic heart disease (IHD) and stroke. While IHD deaths have increased over time, stroke deaths have decreased. A smaller yet significant proportion of deaths were caused by communicable diseases, especially pneumonia, along with a large number of neonatal and maternal deaths. Injuries accounted for the smallest proportion, with falls and road traffic injuries being the most common. Over the last 30 years, there has been a general improvement in global health, and there are fewer deaths from communicable disease [1]. As the Socio-Demographic Index has increased worldwide, there has been a shift in the burden of disease from CMNN diseases towards non-communicable diseases (NCDs) between 1990 and 2019. The WHO reported in 2021 that NCDs account for 71% of all global deaths, with 77% of these occurring in low- and middle-income countries [11]. Increased knowledge of disease transmission and prevention, along with better access to medications and vaccines, has significantly reduced the burden of communicable diseases.

2.7   Global DALYs

This figure highlights the global DALYs and age-standardised DALY rates between 1990 and 2019. During this time, the number of global DALYs has remained constant. However, the age-standardised DALY rates (which take into consideration population growth and the ageing population effects) have reduced during this time. This indicates a great improvement in the overall health of the population (Fig. 2.1).

2.8   Age-Related Trends

Between 1990 and 2019, there was an increase in Disability-Adjusted Life Years (DALYs) among the older population. The six diseases and injuries contributing to this increased burden include ischaemic heart disease, diabetes, stroke, chronic kidney disease, lung cancer and age-related hearing loss. In contrast, in the younger population, the increased burden of disease from DALYs related to HIV/AIDS, musculoskeletal disorders, low back pain and depression. Of these, only HIV/AIDS, musculoskeletal disorders, and diabetes experienced increases in age-standardised DALY rates from 2009 to 2019, with increases of 58.5%, 30.7%, and 24.4%, respectively. A peak in the burden of disease was seen in 2004 due to HIV/AIDS but has

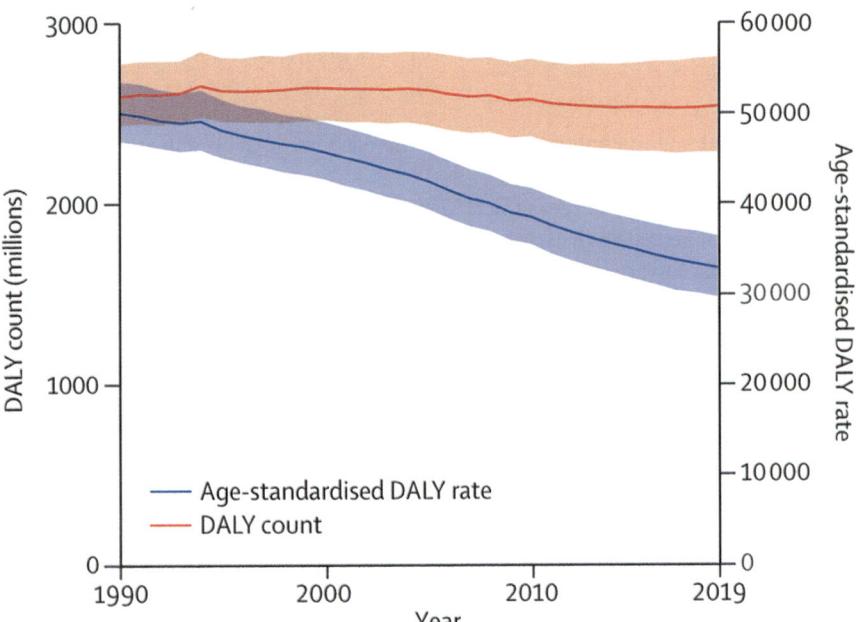

Fig. 2.1 Global DALYs and age-standardised DALY rates, 1990–2019 [1]

A All ages

Leading causes 1990	Percentage of DALYs 1990	Leading causes 2019	Percentage of DALYs 2019	Percentage change in number of DALYs, 1990-2019	Percentage change in age-standardised DALY rate, 1990-2019
1 Neonatal disorders	10·6 (9·9 to 11·4)	1 Neonatal disorders	7·3 (6·4 to 8·4)	−32·3 (−41·7 to −20·8)	−32·6 (−42·1 to −21·2)
2 Lower respiratory infections	8·7 (7·6 to 10·0)	2 Ischaemic heart disease	7·2 (6·5 to 7·9)	50·4 (39·9 to 60·2)	−28·6 (−33·3 to −24·2)
3 Diarrhoeal diseases	7·3 (5·9 to 8·8)	3 Stroke	5·7 (5·1 to 6·2)	32·4 (22·0 to 42·2)	−35·2 (−40·5 to −30·5)
4 Ischaemic heart disease	4·7 (4·4 to 5·0)	4 Lower respiratory infections	3·8 (3·3 to 4·3)	−56·7 (−64·2 to −47·5)	−62·5 (−69·0 to −54·9)
5 Stroke	4·2 (3·9 to 4·5)	5 Diarrhoeal diseases	3·2 (2·6 to 4·0)	−57·5 (−66·2 to −44·7)	−64·6 (−71·7 to −54·2)
6 Congenital birth defects	3·2 (2·3 to 4·8)	6 COPD	2·9 (2·6 to 3·2)	25·6 (15·1 to 46·0)	−39·8 (−44·9 to −30·2)
7 Tuberculosis	3·1 (2·8 to 3·4)	7 Road injuries	2·9 (2·6 to 3·0)	2·4 (−6·9 to 10·8)	−31·0 (−37·1 to −25·4)
8 Road injuries	2·7 (2·6 to 3·0)	8 Diabetes	2·8 (2·5 to 3·1)	147·9 (135·9 to 158·9)	24·4 (18·5 to 29·7)
9 Measles	2·7 (0·9 to 5·6)	9 Low back pain	2·5 (1·9 to 3·1)	46·9 (43·3 to 50·5)	−16·3 (−17·1 to −15·5)
10 Malaria	2·5 (1·4 to 4·1)	10 Congenital birth defects	2·1 (1·7 to 2·6)	−37·3 (−50·6 to −12·8)	−40·0 (−52·7 to −17·1)
11 COPD	2·3 (1·9 to 2·5)	11 HIV/AIDS	1·9 (1·6 to 2·2)	127·7 (97·3 to 171·7)	58·5 (37·1 to 89·2)
12 Protein-energy malnutrition	2·0 (1·6 to 2·7)	12 Tuberculosis	1·9 (1·7 to 2·0)	−41·0 (−47·2 to −33·5)	−62·8 (−66·6 to −58·0)
13 Low back pain	1·7 (1·2 to 2·1)	13 Depressive disorders	1·8 (1·4 to 2·4)	61·1 (56·9 to 65·0)	−1·8 (−2·9 to −0·8)
14 Self-harm	1·4 (1·2 to 1·5)	14 Malaria	1·8 (0·9 to 3·1)	−29·4 (−56·9 to 6·6)	−37·8 (−61·9 to −6·2)
15 Cirrhosis	1·3 (1·2 to 1·5)	15 Headache disorders	1·8 (0·4 to 3·8)	56·7 (52·4 to 62·1)	1·1 (−4·2 to 2·9)
16 Meningitis	1·3 (1·1 to 1·5)	16 Cirrhosis	1·8 (1·6 to 2·0)	33·0 (22·4 to 48·2)	−26·8 (−32·5 to −19·0)
17 Drowning	1·3 (1·1 to 1·4)	17 Lung cancer	1·8 (1·6 to 2·0)	69·1 (53·1 to 85·4)	−16·2 (−24·0 to −8·2)
18 Headache disorders	1·1 (0·2 to 2·4)	18 Chronic kidney disease	1·6 (1·5 to 1·8)	93·2 (81·6 to 105·0)	6·3 (0·2 to 12·4)
19 Depressive disorders	1·1 (0·8 to 1·5)	19 Other musculoskeletal	1·6 (1·2 to 2·1)	128·9 (122·0 to 136·3)	30·7 (27·6 to 34·3)
20 Diabetes	1·1 (1·0 to 1·2)	20 Age-related hearing loss	1·6 (1·2 to 2·1)	87·8 (75·2 to 88·9)	−1·8 (−3·7 to −0·1)
21 Lung cancer	1·0 (1·0 to 1·1)	21 Falls	1·5 (1·4 to 1·7)	47·1 (31·5 to 61·0)	−14·5 (−22·5 to −7·4)
22 Falls	1·0 (0·9 to 1·2)	22 Self-harm	1·3 (1·2 to 1·5)	−5·6 (−14·2 to 3·7)	−38·9 (−44·3 to −33·0)
23 Dietary iron deficiency	1·0 (0·7 to 1·3)	23 Gynaecological diseases	1·2 (0·9 to 1·5)	48·7 (45·8 to 51·8)	−6·8 (−8·7 to −4·9)
24 Interpersonal violence	0·9 (0·9 to 1·0)	24 Anxiety disorders	1·1 (0·8 to 1·5)	53·7 (48·8 to 59·1)	−0·1 (−1·0 to 0·7)
25 Whooping cough	0·9 (0·4 to 1·7)	25 Dietary iron deficiency	1·1 (0·8 to 1·5)	13·8 (10·5 to 17·2)	−16·4 (−18·7 to −14·0)
27 Age-related hearing loss	0·8 (0·6 to 1·1)	26 Interpersonal violence	1·1 (1·0 to 1·2)	10·2 (3·2 to 19·2)	−23·8 (−28·6 to −17·8)
29 Chronic kidney disease	0·8 (0·8 to 0·9)	40 Meningitis	0·6 (0·5 to 0·8)	−51·3 (−59·4 to −42·0)	−57·2 (−64·4 to −48·6)
30 HIV/AIDS	0·8 (0·6 to 1·0)	41 Protein-energy malnutrition	0·6 (0·5 to 0·7)	−71·1 (−79·6 to −59·7)	−74·5 (−82·0 to −64·5)
32 Gynaecological diseases	0·8 (0·6 to 1·0)	46 Drowning	0·5 (0·5 to 0·6)	−60·6 (−65·2 to −53·6)	−68·2 (−71·9 to −62·8)
34 Anxiety disorders	0·7 (0·5 to 1·0)	55 Whooping cough	0·4 (0·2 to 0·7)	−54·5 (−74·6 to −16·9)	−56·3 (−75·6 to −20·3)
35 Other musculoskeletal	0·7 (0·5 to 1·0)	71 Measles	0·3 (0·1 to 0·6)	−89·8 (−92·3 to −86·8)	−90·4 (−92·8 to −87·5)

▇	Communicable, maternal, neonatal and nutritional diseases
▇	Non-communicable diseases
▇	Injuries
—	Increase in rank
- - -	Decrease in rank

Fig. 2.2 Causes of global DALYs, percentage of total DALYs (1990 and 2019), percentage change in number of DALYs and age-standardised DALY rates from 1990 to 2019 for both sexes combined for all ages [1]

since declined significantly due to the increase in use of anti-retroviral therapy (ART).

The most substantial decrease in DALYs, and thus, burden of disease, from 1990 to 2019 was observed in diseases primarily affecting children. These include diarrhoeal diseases, lower respiratory infections, congenital birth defects, neonatal disorders, measles, protein-energy malnutrition, malaria and drowning. Additionally, the burden of tuberculosis, which affects individuals of all ages, also decreased during this period. This reduction in DALYs is reflected in a lower age-standardised DALY rate for these conditions (Fig. 2.2).

2.9 National Trends

The heat map illustrates the DALYs from non-communicable disease and injuries in 1990 (A) compared to 2019 (B). Overall, we see an increase in the number of Years Lived with Disability (YLD), which contributes to increased DALYs over

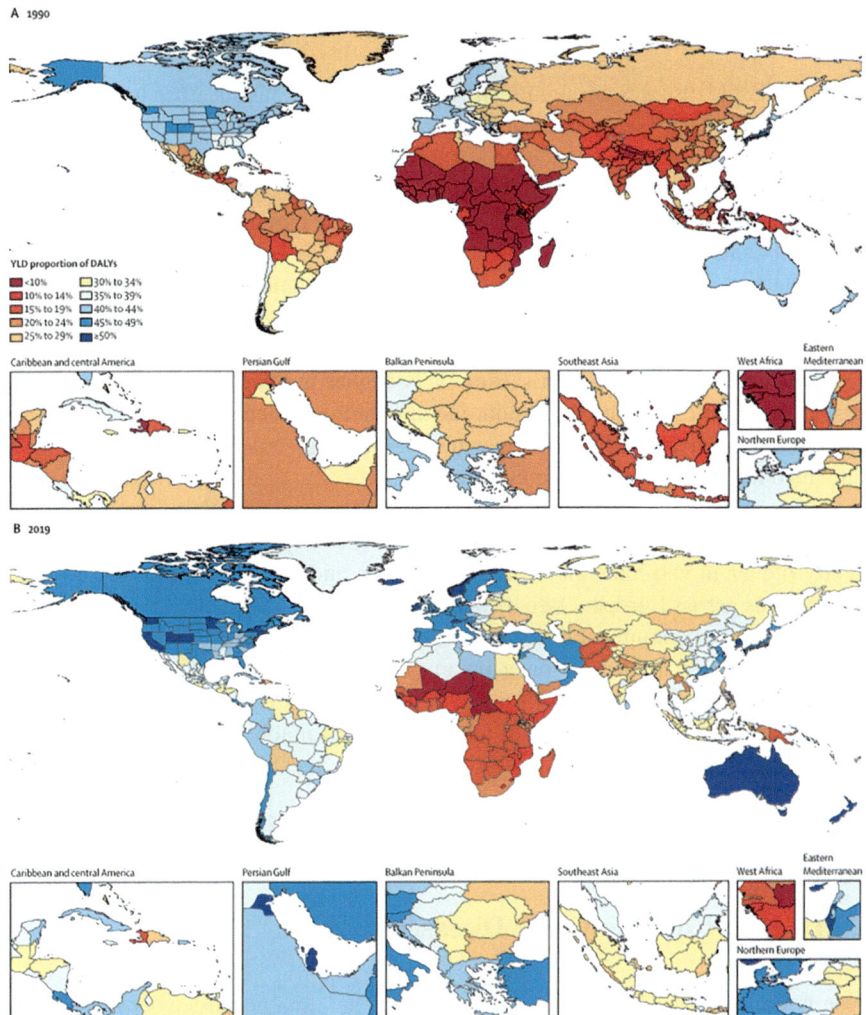

Fig. 2.3 Proportion of total DALYs contributed by injury and non-communicable disease YLDs, by country or territory, 1990 (**a**) and 2019 (**b**) [1]

this time. In 2019, non-communicable disease and injury accounted for > 50% of total DALYs in 11 countries. These are mostly high SDI countries, including Australia, New Zealand, USA, Iceland, Norway, Switzerland and South-East Asia. This figure underscores the growing burden of disability, with significant contributors being musculoskeletal disorders and mental health disorders (Fig. 2.3).

2.10   CMNN Diseases

Communicable diseases are significantly more likely to cause death in low- resource countries where they represent a major burden of disease. Poor sanitation, cramped living spaces and poor education on sexual health contribute to the rapid spread of disease. In contrast, countries with more resources implement measures to reduce transmission, making communicable diseases a lesser burden on healthcare systems in middle- and high-income nations [10].

While communicable disease continues to pose a significant challenge, there has been a steep reduction in the number of deaths from communicable diseases in the last 30 years in lower-income countries [13]. Nevertheless, mortality rates from communicable diseases remain substantially higher in low-resource settings compared to wealthier nations. In middle-income nations, death rates from communicable diseases have reduced slightly, while in higher-income nations, the rates have remained largely stable over the last 30 years.

Lower respiratory tract infections are a leading cause of death by communicable diseases. Although these infections are common globally, mortality rates are significantly higher in sub-Saharan Africa, South Asia and South America than in high SDI nations across Europe, Oceania and North America [10, 13].

In addition to communicable diseases, maternal and neonatal mortality is a significant burden of disease in lower-income nations. Maternal and neonatal deaths account for a large proportion of deaths in the CMNN category. This is due to a range of factors including a lack of resources and available services to allow pregnant people to give birth safely, as well as a lack of education about accessing medical attention during labour [14].

2.11   Non-Communicable Diseases

Non-communicable diseases are more likely to be a major burden for higher SDI nations. This is because higher SDI countries have often put in place strategies to control the transmission of CMNN diseases and have safer maternity care, and populations tend to live in safer, less cramped housing with access to safe water. Higher-income countries often have ageing populations who are more susceptible to developing chronic conditions such as ischaemic heart disease, cancer and dementia later in life. Furthermore, many lifestyle factors prevalent in higher-income countries, such as sedentary lifestyles, poor diet and smoking, increase the likelihood of developing various non-communicable conditions [11]. In recent years, deaths from non-communicable diseases have increased slightly in higher SDI nations, while medium SDI nations have seen an even steeper rise. This is attributed to improved healthcare causing longer lifespans and a higher prevalence of chronic disease. In lower SDI nations, rates of mortality from non-communicable diseases have remained relatively steady in the last few decades [13]. As low-income countries continue to develop, it is possible that these trends may change.

Cardiovascular disease is a major cause of death by non-communicable disease. There are particularly high rates in middle-income and higher-income nations in Eastern Europe, and particularly low rates in low-income nations in Africa and South America. High rates of cardiovascular disease are also observed in North America and Central Asia. [13]. Therefore, this shows a distinct increased burden for these diseases in wealthier nations. This could be due to an ageing population, lack of communicable diseases and the increased unhealthy lifestyle choices due to increased wealth.

2.12 Injuries

Deaths have gradually decreased from injuries in all countries, but particularly in low and middle SDI countries. In 2019, the rates of injury-related deaths were similar across all SDI categories, with higher SDI nations experiencing stable rates that are generally lower than those in middle- and lower-SDI countries. However, there have been more significant reductions in deaths from injuries in middle and lower SDI nations in recent years than in high SDI nations [13].

Motor vehicle road crashes accounted for the highest deaths of any mortality from an injury. They were particularly high in Saudi Arabia, Oman, Central African Republic and South Africa. Saudi Arabia and Oman are examples of high-income countries, South Africa a middle-income and Central African Republic a low-income country [13]. This illustrates the influence of geographical and social factors on deaths, alongside income. This could be due to the increased urbanisation and development in high-income countries. The 'rat race' of developed society translates to high vehicle density on the roads and long traffic queues [15]. Croatia, France, Finland and Norway all have high rates of deaths from falls [13]. This trend can be explained by the ageing populations of these high SDI countries, resulting in an increased risk of non-communicable diseases, chronic diseases and comorbidity. In contrast, in low SDI countries, the lower fall rates are in keeping with their younger populations who have lower life expectancies and are therefore unlikely to ever develop these NCDs [11, 12].

Another interesting pattern seen is a significant increase in deaths associated with natural disasters, particularly in low and middle SDI countries [13]. This highlights their vulnerability within some of these impoverished communities, highlighting their difficulties in recovering physically and economically from such events.

2.13   Burden of Disease Comparison

2.13.1   What Are the Burdens of Disease in Low Socio-Demographic Index Countries?

As stated previously, low SDI countries experience higher rates of death from communicable disease and maternal and neonatal death, although fatalities from non-communicable diseases are also on the rise. The types of communicable diseases prevalent in low SDI countries also differ greatly from those seen in high SDI countries. Furthermore, certain injuries are more common in low SDI countries, such as natural disasters, conflict and violence. The table below explains some risk factors for the most common causes of death in lower SDI countries (Table 2.4).

2.13.2   What Are the Burdens of Middle Socio-Demographic Index Countries?

The burden of disease in middle SDI countries shows a shift towards non-communicable diseases compared to low SDI countries. There has been an increase in deaths from non-communicable diseases in recent years, while the opposite trend is observed for communicable diseases, with the exception of HIV. Furthermore, injuries make up a greater proportion of the deaths in middle SDI countries than low-resource countries, with falls, road injuries and self-harm being the leading causes of death within this category (Table 2.5).

Table 2.4 Causes of communicable disease and risk factors

Diseases in low SDI countries	Risk factors
Diarrhoea	Unsafe drinking water, poor sewerage, poor hygiene
Lower respiratory infections	Lack of vaccinations
HIV	Lack of access to sexual health education and regular HIV testing
Neonatal	Premature birth, low birth weight, intrapartum asphyxiation, antepartum haemorrhage

[10, 14, 16]

2.13.3   What Are the Burdens of High Socio-Demographic Index Countries?

In high SDI countries, the cause of deaths is highest from non-communicable diseases, rather than CMNN diseases or injuries. The main diseases affecting high SDI countries are:

- IHD
- Stroke
- Lung cancer
- Alzheimer's
- Colorectal cancer

Most of the diseases in these countries are preventable by tackling modifiable risk factors. The main factors influencing a high socio-demographic index country include urbanisation, development and globalisation [15]. Increased wealth has led to differences in diets and lifestyle, causing increased consumption of fast-food and saturated fats and a lack of physical activity. These are major factors for developing obesity, hypertension and hypercholesterolemia, which all increase the risk of non-communicable diseases in these countries including IHD and strokes [11]. As these countries become wealthier, life expectancy increases, creating an ageing population. This increases the risk for developing several other non-communicable diseases including Alzheimer's disease, cardiorespiratory disease and cancers [17].

With the high prevalence of dementia and Alzheimer's disease in the over 75 age group, there has been an increase in falls. This demonstrates the need to invest in research to develop better treatments for this disease but also to address other risk factors, including tobacco use, physical inactivity and hearing loss. The increased risk of falls may also be linked to psychotropic and cardiovascular medications, cognitive impairment, depression and general frailty. To mitigate this issue, there is a need for education of the elderly and encouragement of exercise. Occupational therapy teams can also make a difference by providing home safety modifications [19].

In high SDI countries, deaths have also increased from drug abuse, especially in the United States of America. Contributing factors are the over-prescribing of

Table 2.5 Common diseases and risk factors in middle income nations

Commonest diseases in middle SDI countries	Risk factors
Alzheimer's	Old age, inactivity, smoking, vascular disease (hypertension, hypercholesterolemia), genetics
Cancer	Smoking, older age, poor diet
Road injury	Improper use of seatbelts, unsafe roads, unqualified drivers, lack of safe pedestrian spaces
TB	HIV, diabetes, immunosuppression, smoking, alcohol use

[10, 12, 15, 17, 18]

high-dose opioids, inadequate opioid substitution therapy and the increasing incidence of street drugs laced with highly potent opioids such as fentanyl [1].

There is a significant burden from lung cancer and COPD, which are more prevalent from age 50 and above. This is due to the risk factors of increased tobacco use and air pollution. To reduce air pollution, strategies like encouraging greener transport, more green spaces within cities and reducing the emissions of greenhouse gases could be implemented. Occupational hazards like asbestos have also been seen to contribute to lung cancer and mesotheliomas, highlighting the need for stricter occupational regulations and monitoring [1, 11].

2.14   Reducing the Burden of Disease

Here, we propose possible strategies to reduce the burden of disease specific to a country's stage of development and economic status (Table 2.6):

Table 2.6 Solutions to reduce burden of disease by income level

Low SDI countries	Middle SDI countries	High SDI countries
Investing in clean water pumps for villages and toilets with proper waste disposal	Legislation on the selling of tobacco products	Legislation on the selling and use of tobacco
Improved vaccination programmes	Education on healthy diet choices	Legislation on the selling and use of alcohol
Improved access to antibiotics and other basic healthcare	Safer roads and higher vehicle safety standards	Tighter occupational safety regulations
Sexual health education and improved contraceptive availability	Designated pedestrian areas	Sexual health education
Improved antenatal care and higher-level training for healthcare workers	Speed limits and legislation on seat belts	Better access to barrier methods of contraception
Formal education for women and girls	Better access to barrier methods and contraception and HIV tests	Reducing air pollution

2.15   Evaluation of the GBD Database

Strengths of the GBD Database:

- Improvement in data collection and analysis methods
- Public availability and accessibility of data
- Study over a long period of time
- Reliable publishers—The WHO, IHME, The Lancet
- 204 countries and 369 diseases—worldwide data
- High SDI countries have more accurate ways to collect primary data

Limitations of the GBD Database:

- Lack of availability of primary data—predictions were made
- Low SDI country might not have the preferred method of collecting data
- Broad categorisation of diseases
- Doesn't consider comorbidity
- Doesn't account for regional differences between a country
- Doesn't classify all diseases that exist
- Confidentiality and willingness of people to share health-related information

References

1. Vos T, Lim SS, Abbafati C, Abbas KM, Abbasi M, Abbasifard M, et al. Global burden of 369 diseases and injuries in 204 countries and territories, 1990–2019: a systematic analysis for the Global Burden of Disease Study 2019. The Lancet. 2020;396:1135–59. https://doi.org/10.1016/S0140-6736(20)30925-9.
2. World Health Organization. Disability-adjusted life years (DALYs). 2023 [accessed 23 June 2023]. Available from: https://www.who.int/data/gho/indicator-metadata-registry/imr-details/158
3. World Health Organization. Years of healthy life lost due to disability (YLD). 2023 [accessed 23 June 2023]. Available from: https://www.who.int/data/gho/indicator-metadata-registry/imr-details/160
4. World Health Organization. International Statistical Classification of Diseases and Related Health Problems (ICD). 2021 [accessed 23 June 2023]. Available at: https://www.who.int/standards/classifications/classification-of-diseases
5. Institute for Health Metrics and Evaluation. Socio-demographic Index (SDI). 2023 [accessed 23 June 2023]. Available at: https://www.healthdata.org/taxonomy/glossary/socio-demographic-index-sdi
6. The World Bank. Classifying countries by income. 2019 [accessed 23 June 2023]. Available at: https://datatopics.worldbank.org/world-development-indicators/stories/the-classification-of-countries-by-income.html
7. Global Health Data Exchange. Global Burden of Disease Study 2019 (GBD 2019) Socio-Demographic Index (SDI) 1950-2019. 2023 [accessed 23 June 2023]. Available at: https://ghdx.healthdata.org/record/ihme-data/gbd-2019-socio-demographic-index-sdi-1950-2019
8. Institute for Health Metrics and Evaluation. A new way of measuring development helps assess health system performance. 2017 [accessed 23 June 2023]. Available at: https://www.healthdata.org/acting-data/new-way-measuring-development-helps-assess-health-system-performance

9. World Health Organization. Social determinants of health. 2023 [accessed 23 June 2023]. Available at: https://www.who.int/health-topics/social-determinants-of-health#tab=tab_1

10. World Health Organization. Communicable and noncommunicable diseases, and mental health. 2023 [accessed 23 June 2023]. Available at: https://www.who.int/our-work/communicable-and-noncommunicable-diseases-and-mental-health

11. World Health Organization. Noncommunicable diseases. 2022 [accessed 23 June 2023]. Available at: https://www.who.int/news-room/fact-sheets/detail/noncommunicable-diseases

12. World Health Organization/Injuries and violence. 2021 [accessed 23 June 2023]. Available at: https://www.who.int/news-room/fact-sheets/detail/injuries-and-violence

13. The Lancet. GBD Compare. 2019 [accessed 23 June 2023]. Available at: https://www.thelancet.com/lancet/visualisations/gbd-compare

14. World Health Organization. Maternal and newborn health. 2010 [accessed 23 June 2023]. Available at: https://www.who.int/europe/news-room/fact-sheets/item/maternal-and-newborn-health

15. World Health Organization. Urban health. 2021 [accessed 23 June 2023]. Available at: https://www.who.int/news-room/fact-sheets/detail/urban-health#:~:text=Urbanization%20is%20also%20linked%20to%20high%20rates%20of,and%20a%20lack%20of%20safe%20transport%20and%20infrastructure

16. Centers for Disease Control and Prevention. Disease Threats and Global WASH Killers: Cholera, Typhoid, and Other Waterborne Infections. 2020 [accessed 23 June 2023]. Available at: https://www.cdc.gov/healthywater/global/WASH.html?CDC_AA_refVal=https%3A%2F%2Fwww.cdc.gov%2Fhealthywater%2Fglobal%2Fdiarrhea-burden.html

17. Alzheimer's Research UK. Risk factors. 2022 [accessed 23 June 2023]. Available at: https://www.alzheimersresearchuk.org/dementia-information/types-of-dementia/alzheimers-disease/risk-factors/

18. Centers for Disease Control and Prevention. TB Risk Factors. 2016 [accessed 23 June 2023]. Available at: https://www.cdc.gov/tb/topic/basics/risk.htm

19. Kato-Narita EM, Radanovic M. Characteristics of falls in mild and moderate Alzheimer's disease. Dement Neuropsychol. 2009;3(4):337–43. https://doi.org/10.1590/S1980-57642009DN30400013.

Chapter 3
Changing Demographics and Disease Burden in Low Resource Countries

Giovanna Giona, Lauren Cooper, and Abi Butt

3.1 Socio-Economic Determinants of Health

Many factors contribute to the health of individuals and populations. These can be social and economic factors, the physical environment and an individual's characteristics and behaviours (refer to Fig. 3.1) [1].

Socio-economic determinants of health also include the availability and accessibility of healthcare, employment, education, food and housing. Additionally, examples include an individual's gender, age and the conditions in which they live.

These factors are often influenced by a country's society and government, which oversee the distribution of these basic resources. Therefore, they are subject to change. This helps to explain the variation observed in global health and demographics, as observed by the World Health Organisation [2].

Health inequity exists in all countries, including higher-income countries, where certain barriers may hinder individuals in these populations from accessing the

G. Giona (✉) · L. Cooper · A. Butt
School of Medicine, Cardiff University, Cardiff, UK

A. Fiander, G. Fry (eds.), *A Healthcare Students Introduction to Global Health*, https://doi.org/10.1007/978-3-031-66563-9_3

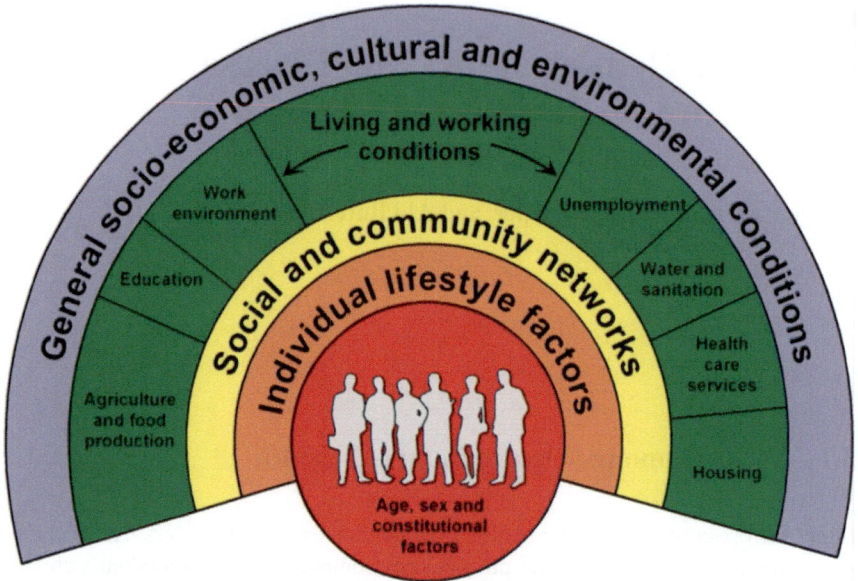

Fig. 3.1 The Dahlgren and Whitehead model of health determinants [3]

necessary healthcare. Poor health is often associated with underlying socio-economic disadvantages [4].

3.2 Demographics

Epidemiology is the study of the distribution and determinants, causes and risk factors, of health-related states and events in specified populations and the application of this study to the control of health problems' [5, 6].

International Classification of Diseases (ICD)
ICD is the global health information standard for mortality and morbidity statistics.

It is used in clinical care and research to define diseases and study disease patterns, manage health care, monitor outcomes and allocate resources.

More than 100 countries use ICD to report mortality data which is a primary indicator of health status abd therefore allows worldwide monitoring including the progress toward the Sustainable Development Goals [7].

Epidemiological data can be used to explore the causes of health outcomes and diseases within populations; plan and evaluate strategies to prevent illness and guide the management of patients in whom the disease has already developed.

3.3 Disease Burden in Low Resource Countries

There has been a recent shift in terms of the burden of disease in LRCs. Where communicable, maternal, neonatal and nutritional diseases (CMNN) once contributed the greatest burden of disease, these have been superseded by non-communicable diseases (NCDs). In 2019, NCDs caused 71% of global deaths [8].

Communicable Diseases
Can be transferred from one person to another, or from one organism to another. Examples include measles, malaria and human immunosuppressive virus (HIV).

Non-Communicable Diseases
Cannot be transferred between people or other organisms. Examples include cardiovascular diseases, types of cancer or dementia [9].

There are several reasons for this shift. Most importantly, due to advances in the research of communicable diseases, including the significant emphasis on promoting adequate hygiene, administering vaccinations against preventable diseases and utilising antibiotic treatments [10].

  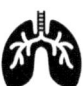

There has also been rapidly evolving research into implementing preventative and curative measures towards non-communicable diseases, such as cancer [11].

Moreover, there has been an increased global awareness and global education regarding the impacts of unhealthy lifestyle choices and the prevention of chronic disease. These include campaigns against smoking, excessive alcohol consumption, high saturated fat and salt intake and an insufficient intake of fruit and vegetables.

3.4   Global Incidence of Communicable Diseases

Communicable diseases continue to be a significant burden to low resource countries despite the global shift towards NCDs, subsequently affecting the mortality of a low resource country (LRC). This burden can be measured in Disability-Adjusted Life Years (DALYs) which equates to one lost year of healthy life (see Fig. 3.2). For example, in Central African Republic, an LRC, there were 50,790.26 per 100,000 DALYs compared to a significantly lower number of 1380.85 per 100,000 in the United Kingdom, a high resource country (HRC). This supports current evidence of relationships between socio-economic determinants of health and health outcomes. For example, basic public health measures and resources, such as access to clean water, adequate hygiene and accessible healthcare services, explain some of these discrepancies.

Similarly, there is a strong negative correlation between a country's gross domestic product (GDP) per capita and the disease burden due to communicable diseases (see Fig. 3.3). For example, LRCs such as Zimbabwe and Ghana, with a lower GDP per capita, have a higher number of DALYs due to communicable diseases. In contrast, HRCs with a higher GDP per capita, such as the United States, United Kingdom and Australia, have fewer DALYs and disease burden.

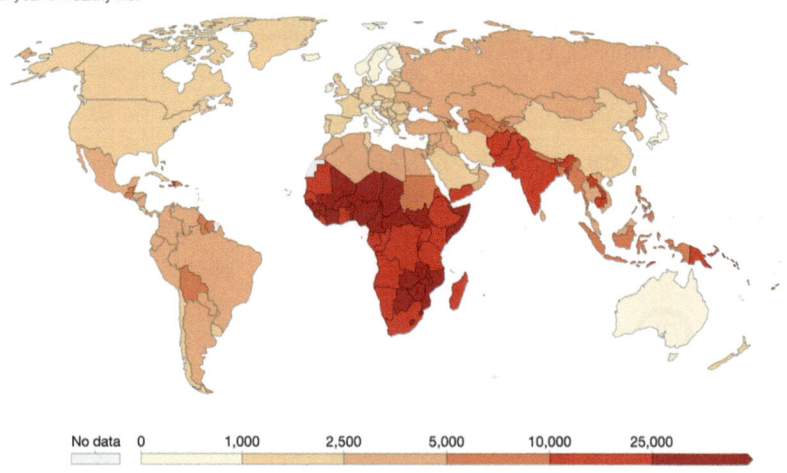

DALY rates from communicable, neonatal, maternal & nutritional diseases, 2019

Our World in Data

Age-standardized DALY (Disability-Adjusted Life Year) rates per 100,000 individuals from communicable diseases. DALYs are used to measure total burden of disease - both from years of life lost and years lived with a disability. One DALY equals one lost year of healthy life.

No data   0   1,000   2,500   5,000   10,000   25,000

Source: IHME, Global Burden of Disease   CC BY

Fig. 3.2 Visual illustration of the disability-adjusted life year (DALY) rates, used to measure the burden from communicable, maternal, neonatal and nutritional diseases, by country in 2019, whereby one DALY equates to one lost year of healthy life [12]

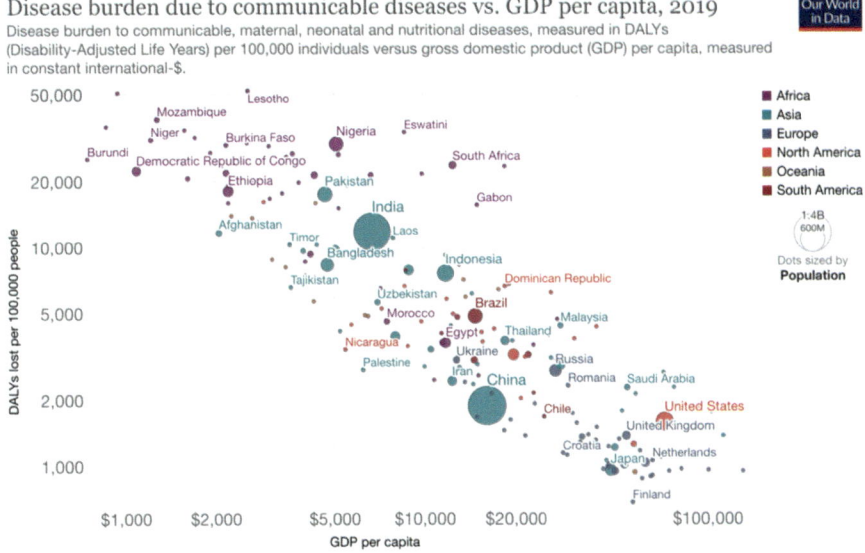

Fig. 3.3 The relationship between communicable disease burden and gross domestic product (GDP) per capita by country [12, 13]

3.5 Global Incidence of Non-Communicable Diseases

Non-communicable diseases that were once considered an issue for HRCs are now increasing in prevalence in LRCs too. The change in overall disease patterns means that there will need to be greater emphasis on tackling chronic disease in the future [14, 15].

This poses a host of implications on LRCs. For example, to effectively treat NCDs, more patients would need to be treated in a primary setting. This would mean a higher demand for remote health clinics and specialist health services [14, 15]. This requires more funding, infrastructure, training and staff, all of which are often lacking in LRCs.

Furthermore, NCDs also present an added burden to society [14, 15]. For example, chronic illness may lead to increased time off work, which affects the overall economy, family dynamics and personal quality of life. Moreover, many NCDs are treated pharmacologically. For example, metformin treats diabetes, statins treat increased cholesterol and ACE inhibitors treat hypertension. This requires increased costs for transportation to obtain medication, finances, storage facilities and overall, a greater reliance on the healthcare system of the country.

Are LRCs equipped with the staff and resources to handle this shift? Will it overwhelm their already under-resourced healthcare systems?

References

1. GOV.UK. Chapter 6: social determinants of health [Internet]. 2017 [cited 2020 Nov 12]. Available from: https://www.gov.uk/government/publications/health-profile-for-england/chapter-6-social-determinants-of-health
2. World Health Organisation. Social determinants of health: Key concepts [Internet]. 2013 [cited 2020 Nov 10]. Available from: https://www.who.int/news-room/q-a-detail/social-determinants-of-health-key-concepts
3. Eikemo, T. et al. The first pan-European sociological health inequalities survey of the general population: the European social survey rotating module on the social determinants of health [Internet]. 2016 [cited 2020 Nov 12];33 (1), pp. 137–153. Available from: https://academic.oup.com/esr/article/33/1/137/2525456
4. Orach CG. Health equity: challenges in low-income countries. African health sciences [Internet]. 2009 [cited 2020 Nov 10]; 9(2), pp. S49–S51. Available from: https://pubmed.ncbi.nlm.nih.gov/20589106/
5. Kesteloot, H. Epidemiology: past, present and future. Verhandelingen – Koninklijke Academie voor Geneeskunde van Belgie [Internet]. 2004 [cited 2020 Nov 10]; 66(5–6), pp. 384–405. Available from: https://pubmed.ncbi.nlm.nih.gov/15641567/
6. Coggon D What is epidemiology? [Internet]. 2004 [cited 2020 Nov 11]. Available from: https://www.bmj.com/about-bmj/resources-readers/publications/epidemiology-uninitiated/1-what-epidemiology
7. World Health Organisation. International Classification of Diseases (ICD) Information Sheet [Internet]. 2017 [cited 2020 Nov 11]. Available at: https://www.who.int/classifications/icd/factsheet/en/
8. Bigna JJ, Noubiap JJ. The rising burden of non-communicable diseases in sub-Saharan Africa. The Lancet Global Health [Internet]. 2019 [cited 2020 Nov 10]; 7(10), pp. e1295–e1296. Available from: https://www.thelancet.com/pdfs/journals/langlo/PIIS2214-109X(19)30370-5.pdf
9. Sapkota A Communicable vs non-communicable diseases – definition, 17 differences, examples [Internet]. 2022 [cited 2022 April 19]. Available from: https://microbenotes.com/communicable-vs-non-communicable-diseases/
10. World Health Organisation. Disease and injury country estimates: burden of disease [Internet]. 2008 [cited 2020 Nov 10]. Available from: http://www.who.int/healthinfo/global_burden_disease/estimates_country/en/index.html
11. Centers for Disease Control and Prevention. Historical Evolution of Epidemiology [Internet]. 2012 [cited 2022 April 18]. Available from: https://www.cdc.gov/csels/dsepd/ss1978/lesson1/section2.html
12. Ritchie H, Roser M. Burden of disease. Our world in data [Internet]. 2021 [cited 2022 April 19]. Available from: https://ourworldindata.org/burden-of-disease
13. World Health Organisation. Gross Domestic Product (GDP), per capita, international $ (PPP-adjusted) [Internet]. 2020 [cited 2020 Nov 11]. Available from: https://www.who.int/data/gho/indicator-metadata-registry/imr-details/1145
14. Forouzanfar MH, et al. Global, regional, and national comparative risk assessment of 79 behavioural, environmental and occupational, and metabolic risks or clusters of risks, 19vancou90-2015: a systematic analysis for the Global Burden of Disease Study 2015. The Lancet [Internet]. 2016 [cited 2020 Nov 10]; 388(10053), pp. 1659–1724. Available from: https://pubmed.ncbi.nlm.nih.gov/27733284/
15. World Health Organisation. Global health risks [Internet]. 2009 [cited 2020 Nov 11]. Available from: https://www.who.int/healthinfo/global_burden_disease/GlobalHealthRisks_report_full.pdf

Chapter 4
Urbanisation and Implications for Health

Hozaifa Sahi, Joe O'Connor, Alison Fiander, and Grace Fry

4.1   What Is Urbanisation?

Urbanisation can be defined as an increase in the population of urban areas with a concurrent decrease in the population in rural areas. Recent decades have witnessed a dramatic, rapid increase in urbanisation. Between 1950 and 2018, the proportion of the population living in urbanised areas grew from 30% to 55% [1]. According to this trend, it is predicted that 68% of individuals will live in urban areas by 2050. There is considerable geographical variation in the rate of urbanisation, with developing countries experiencing the greatest rate. Ninety per cent of the projected growth in urbanisation by 2050 will be seen in the Asian and African continents. India, China and Nigeria combined are expected to account for 35% of the growth in the world's urban population between 2018 and 2050.

When it comes to health, urbanisation has both advantages and disadvantages. The complex, inter-dimensional organisation of urban areas means dysfunction in one sector (e.g. government) can have devastating effects on the others (e.g. healthcare) (Fig. 4.1).

H. Sahi (✉) · J. O'Connor · G. Fry
School of Medicine, Cardiff University, Cardiff, UK
e-mail: oconnorj8@cardiff.ac.uk

A. Fiander
Emeritus Chair Obstetrics and Gynaecology, School of Medicine,
Cardiff University, Cardiff, UK
e-mail: fianderan@cf.ac.uk

© The Author(s), under exclusive license to Springer Nature
Switzerland AG 2024
A. Fiander, G. Fry (eds.), *A Healthcare Students Introduction to Global Health*,
https://doi.org/10.1007/978-3-031-66563-9_4

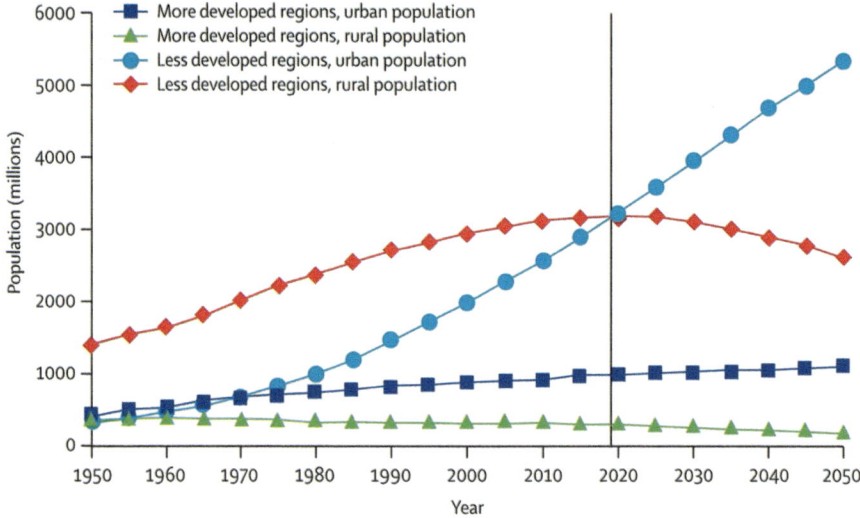

Fig. 4.1 Graph to show the evolution of rural and urban populations between 1950 and 2050 [2]

4.1.1 Evidence for Urbanisation

Urbanisation is on the rise around the world, with 55% of the world's population living in cities in 2018 [1]. By 2050, it's projected that 6.3 billion people globally will live in cities [2].

The phenomenon is most evident in continents with many LRCs, such as Africa. By 2030, it's expected that 50% of Africa's 1 billion inhabitants will live in cities, and the populations of most of these cities are expected to keep growing (Fig. 4.2).

4.2 Reasons for Increasing Urbanisation

The three main causes of increased urbanisation in developing countries are as follows:

1. *Natural Increase of Urban Populations*

   Existing urban populations can grow, independent of migration, when the number of births exceeds the number of deaths in the population. This is due to advancements in healthcare and medical technology which increase life expectancy and improve fertility. Coupled with lower levels of infant mortality, urban populations increase in size.

2. *Rural to Urban Migration*

   Urban populations also increase in size from the movement of people from rural areas into cities. This migratory pattern can be explained by 'push factors' and 'pull factors'.

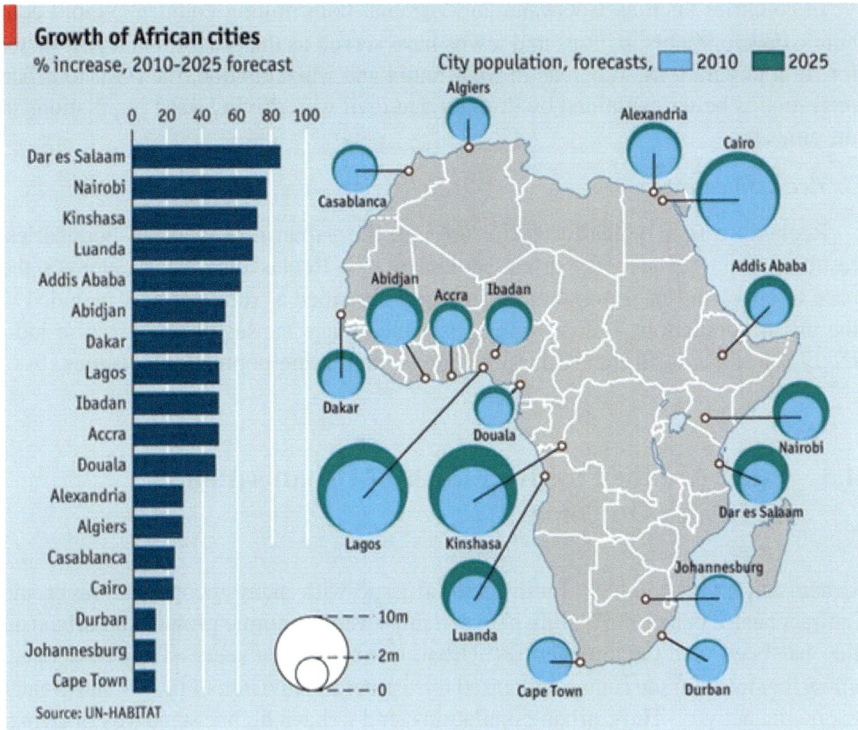

Fig. 4.2 Infographic showing projected population growth of African cities by 2050 [3]

- *Pull Factors:*

Pull factors refer to the aspects of living and working in cities that attract people from more rural areas; these are the factors that give urban life its allure. These include the advantages of the urban lifestyle such as easier access to resources and healthcare, greater employment opportunities and higher income. This in turn increases living standards and health outcomes dramatically, as higher income is strongly associated with better physical and mental health [4]. Furthermore, as urban centres develop and so people and infrastructure become more concentrated, the governmental distribution of healthcare and resources to the population becomes more efficient.

- *Push Factors:*

Push factors refer to those factors that are actively driving people out of rural areas. Whilst urban areas lend themselves to more widespread and even distribution of healthcare and resources, this is more difficult in rural areas due to sparser infrastructure and populations. This leads to people in remote areas having lower life expectancies and higher morbidity, and this disparity is most obvious in LRCs, particularly in Sub-Saharan Africa [5]. Due to their dependence on agriculture as a source of income, rural populations are more financially vulnerable to the effects of climate change and natural disasters. All these factors lead to the phenomenon of rural flight, that is, migration from rural areas.

In countries such as Botswana and Zambia, both mining countries, rapid economic developments in cities and towns have served as the predominant pull factor for rural populations. Whereas in Mauritania and Mozambique, the rural to urban migration is better explained by drought and civil war, driving rural populations to the cities [6].

3. *Reclassification*

Reclassification typically occurs through the expansion of urban boundaries, resulting in larger areas of urban settlement [7]. Reclassification accelerates the pace of urbanisation as populations formerly classified as rural are now included in the urban population. The two previously mentioned causes of urbanisation indirectly contribute to further reclassification by increasing population densities.

4.3   What Are the Positive Effects of Urbanisation on Health Outcomes?

Urbanisation is a complex, multi-factorial issue with many recognised direct and indirect health benefits. The link between improved economic growth and urbanisation has been well documented [8]. Urban settings, when successfully developed, allow for shorter trade routes, increased infrastructure, division of labour and greater economic activity. Thus, urban populations tend to have higher standards of living. Urban areas have been shown to have better access to electricity, clean drinking water and improved sanitation compared to rural areas.

For example, there is a clear relationship between the location of a household, the corresponding level of maternal education and child malnourishment. In more urban locations, the level of maternal education is higher, and there is an associated lower prevalence of childhood stunting [9].

In addition, the establishment of international corporations in urban centres not only provides higher income jobs for workers, but also stimulates other companies and professions in a knock-on multiplier effect, thereby generating greater economic prosperity for the country, which can be used to improve healthcare and infrastructure. This leads to more healthcare professionals being available in urban areas, as shown in a 2017 study which found urban areas have 24.2% more primary care doctors per 100,000 people [10]. This is particularly evident in LRCs, as shown in the figure below which shows the relative availability of various procedures in Nigeria in urban and rural settings [11] (Fig. 4.3).

*Postpartum FP refers to postpartum family planning

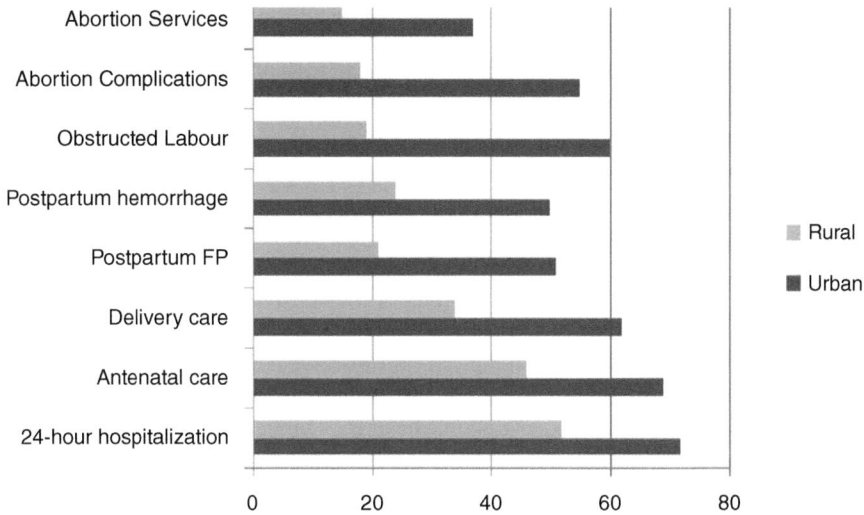

Fig. 4.3 Graph to show the relative availability of maternal healthcare between rural and urban areas in Nigeria [11]

4.4   What Are the Negative Effects of Urbanisation?

Despite the many positives of urbanisation, it does also pose various threats to the health of urban inhabitants. One way is through the development of slums, which are more common in cities in LRCs. The United Nations Human Settlements Programme (UN-HABITAT) defines a slum settlement as a group of individuals living under the same roof in an urban who lack one or more of the following:

Durable housing of a permanent nature that protects against extreme climate conditions.
Sufficient living space, which means no more than three people sharing the same room.
Easy access to safe water in sufficient amounts at an affordable price.
Access to adequate sanitation in the form of a private or public toilet shared by a reasonable number of people.
Security of tenure that prevents forced eviction'.

It is thought that slum development is caused by urbanisation that occurs at an unsustainable rate. Housing construction cannot keep pace with the urban population growth and there is a demand far greater than the city can supply. As a result of this, people end up living in close quarters and in poor conditions. This is associated with a higher mortality rates for children under 5, as well as higher risk of respiratory illness and diarrhoea in children and HIV in adolescents [12].

Furthermore, the urban lifestyle itself may lead to physical health problems. Urban inhabitants do less exercise (due to more sedentary jobs and time spent commuting across large areas) and have less healthy diets (due to the availability of cheap fast and ultra-processed food). This contributes to higher rates of obesity and cardiovascular disease. Also, the effect of air pollution detracts from the positive effects of urbanisation. According to the World Health Organisation, 98% of cities in low–middle-income countries fall short of their air quality guidelines, putting millions at increased risk of various cancers, respiratory illnesses and cardiovascular disease.

Urbanicity impacts mental as well as physical health. The allure of life in the city attracts migrants from different areas and even different countries, isolating individuals from their own family and culture. It is even more difficult to establish social connections in an already overwhelming social environment. This can not only lead to extreme loneliness for many, but also weakens family stability. The effects of this loneliness on the urban setting on physical health shouldn't be underestimated; a study found that lonely people have 26% higher mortality rates, and the effect on their health is equivalent to smoking 15 cigarettes per day [13].

References

1. United Nations. World urbanization prospects: the 2018 revision. 2019. Available at: https://www.un-ilibrary.org/content/books/9789210043144/read
2. Alirol E, Getaz L, Stoll B, Chappuis F, Loutan L. Urbanisation and infectious diseases in a globalised world. Lancet Infect Dis. 2011;11(2):131–41.
3. The Ecomonist. Growth areas. The Ecomonist. 13 Dec 2010. Available at: https://www.economist.com/graphic-detail/2010/12/13/growth-areas
4. Ettner SL. New evidence on the relationship between income and health. J Health Econ. 1996;15(1):67–85.
5. Strasser R, Kam SM, Regalado SM. Rural health care access and policy in developing countries. Annu Rev Public Health. 2016;37:395–412.
6. Godfrey R, Julien M. Urbanisation and health. Clin Med (Lond). 2005;5(2):137–41.
7. Jiang L, O'Neill BC. Determinants of urban growth during demographic and mobility transitions: evidence from India, Mexico, and the US. 2018.
8. Bloom DE, Canning D, Fink G. Urbanization and the wealth of nations. Science. 2008;319(5864):772–5.
9. Cleland JG, Van Ginneken JK. Maternal education and child survival in developing countries: the search for pathways of influence. Soc Sci Med. 1988;27(12):1357–68.
10. North Carolina Rural Health Programme. Rural Health Snapshot. 2017. Available at: https://www.shepscenter.unc.edu/wp-content/uploads/dlm_uploads/2017/05/Snapshot2017.pdf
11. Essien E, Williams EE. E-health services in rural communities in the developing countries. 2nd International Conference on Adaptive Science & Technology (ICAST); 2009 Accra, Ghana. Pages: pp. 218–225. https://doi.org/10.1109/ICASTECH.2009.5409722.
12. Unger A. Children's health in slum settings. Arch Dis Child. 2013;98(10):799–805.
13. Holt-Lunstad J, Smith TB, Baker M, Harris T, Stephenson D. Loneliness and social isolation as risk factors for mortality: a meta-analytic review. Perspect Psychol Sci. 2015;10(2):227–37.

Chapter 5
The Impact of Non-Communicable Diseases in Low- and Middle-Income Countries

Ffyon Davies and Hannah Raval

5.1 What Are NCDs?

Non-communicable diseases (NCDs) are illnesses which cannot be transmitted to others. They are usually chronic conditions with life-long implications. Unlike acute conditions, NCDs progress slowly. They can affect people from anywhere, at any age and are caused by a combination of genetic, physiological, environmental and behavioural factors. NCDs are important to consider in the wider picture of global health, as they are the leading cause of disability and death.

- It is estimated 41 million people die from an NCD worldwide every year, which equates to 74% of deaths globally.
- Approximately 77% of these deaths are in low- and middle-income countries (LMICs), which highlights the inequalities in healthcare across the globe [1] (Fig. 5.1).

F. Davies
Hereford, UK

H. Raval (✉)
School of Medicine, Cardiff University, Cardiff, UK
e-mail: hannah.raval@doctors.org.uk

© The Author(s), under exclusive license to Springer Nature Switzerland AG 2024
A. Fiander, G. Fry (eds.), *A Healthcare Students Introduction to Global Health*,
https://doi.org/10.1007/978-3-031-66563-9_5

Causes of death, World

The estimated annual number of deaths from each broad cause of death: injuries (such as accidents, violence and suicides); communicable, maternal, neonatal and nutritional diseases; and non-communicable diseases[1].

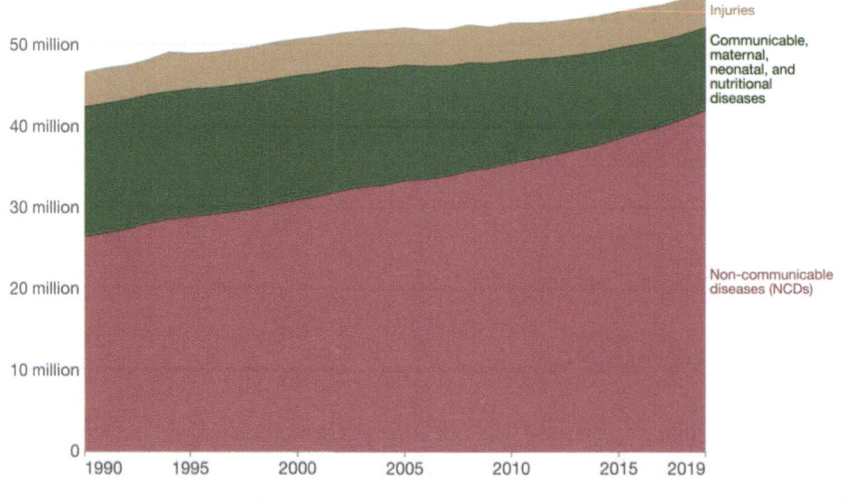

Source: IHME, Global Burden of Disease (2019)   OurWorldInData.org/causes-of-death · CC BY

1. **Non-communicable diseases**: Noncommunicable diseases (NCDs), also known as chronic diseases, tend to be of long duration and are the result of a combination of genetic, physiological, environmental and behavioural factors. The main types of NCD are cardiovascular diseases, cancers, chronic respiratory diseases, and diabetes.

Fig. 5.1 Causes of death, World, 1990–2019 [2]

5.2 Four Main NCDs

- *Cardiovascular disease*—currently the leading cause of death across the globe
- *Cancers*—affecting 9.3 million people globally
- *Chronic respiratory conditions*—such as lung cancer, chronic obstructive pulmonary disease (COPD) and bronchiectasis, many of which are linked to smoking
- *Diabetes*—80% of people living with diabetes are in LMICs [3].

5.3 Other NCDs

- *Mental health problems*—a group of serious conditions which are a leading cause of disability worldwide. Depression in particular is a significant health burden, more commonly affecting women. Mental health conditions are important to consider, as they remain ignored and under-funded, although they represent a huge proportion of health burden and reduce life expectancy. This may be due to stigmatisation of mental health conditions, and education is essential in addressing this.

5.4 Risk Factors

In order to tackle NCDs, healthcare professionals must be familiar with the risk factors contributing to their development. The four main modifiable risk factors include *poor diet*, a *lack of exercise* (typically attributed to urban living), *tobacco* use and *alcohol* consumption. There are some non-modifiable risk factors, such as age or family history, that an individual does not have control over.

5.5 NCDs in LMICs

NCDs affect people worldwide; however, their prevalence and incidence vary from country to country. As discussed previously, this can in part be attributed to differences in lifestyle and behaviour. NCDs have previously been considered diseases of more socio-economically developed countries, countries where risk factors such as access to calorie dense foods are more prevalent. The prevalence of NCDs has risen dramatically in LMICs as economic development has brought with it changes in lifestyle.

The figure below demonstrates how changes related to modernization and economic development in LMICs can lead to a change in lifestyle which promotes NCDs (Fig. 5.2):

As a compounding factor, many people affected by NCDs in LMICs are unable to receive the healthcare treatment they require. This often leads to a greater disease severity, which prevents people from being able to work, resulting in a negative impact on the overall economy. This in turn contributes to overall deprivation and poverty, which drives poor health outcomes in a population, resulting in a cycle of poverty and NCDs (Fig. 5.3).

It is believed that 77% of NCDs deaths occur in LMICs [1]. The WHO has reported that they expect there to be the largest increase in rates of NCDs in the African continent, followed by the Eastern Mediterranean region. They also predict that the greatest number of annual deaths from these diseases will be in the Western Pacific and South-East Asian parts of the world.

Fig. 5.2 Effects of modernization and economic development

Modernization and economic development:
→ Urban lifestyle:
  ➡ change in diet and reduced physical activity
    → increased risk of NCDs related to obesity
  ➡ increased intake of tobacco and alcohol
    → increased risk of NCDs and cancer
  ➡ leads to decline in the birth rate
→ Improved living conditions:
  ➡ improved water & sanitation
    → reduction in infectious diseases
      → decline in the death rate
        → patients survive to an older age
          → higher risk of NCDs e.g diabetes, CVS disease and cancers

Fig. 5.3 Cycle of poverty
and NCDs

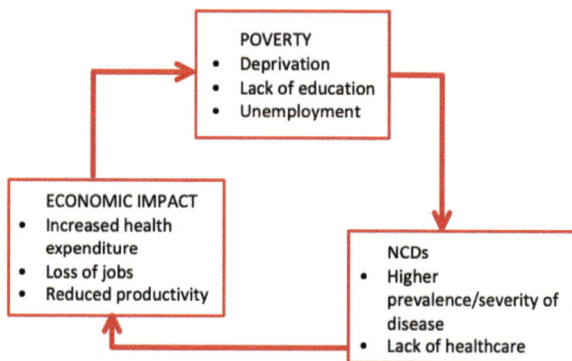

5.6 What Is Epidemiological Transition?

Epidemiological transition is a theory first put forward by Abdel Omran in 1971 [4], which describes a 'complex change in patterns of health and disease and on the interactions between these patterns and their demographic, economic and socio-logic determinants and consequences'. It is a period of development characterised by a sharp increase in population growth rates, due to medical advances in either treatment or prevention of conditions. This phase is then followed by a 'levelling out' phase, due to declines in fertility rates and improvements in medical care that follows. It is this that accounts for change over time, from a high prevalence of infectious disease in a population, to a higher prevalence of chronic disease.

He divided this into several phases, which ultimately leads to chronic disease surpassing infectious disease as the primary cause of death. These phases are:

1. The age of *Pestilence and Famine* = high death rate, low life expectancy.
2. The age of *Receding Pandemics* = death rates decline as pandemics are treated and life expectancy increases steadily, leading to a population growth. Start of shift from infectious diseases to NCDs.
3. The age of *Degeneration and Man-made disease* = death rates decrease and population starts to stabilise, with greatest burden of disease being NCDs (Fig. 5.4).

The Demographic transition model shows the effect of birth and deaths rates on the total population trends. It is divided into 5 phases: high stationary, early expanding, lat expanding, low stationary, declining. The transition between stages occurs as a country develops and modernises its healthcare and public health systems, which can have dramatic effects on birth rates, death rates, infant mortality rates and life expectancy. The transition period is critical in the context of non-communicable diseases, as the country must adapt its healthcare system from being primarily concerned with the control of the spread of infectious epidemics, to long-term care of its chronically ill population.

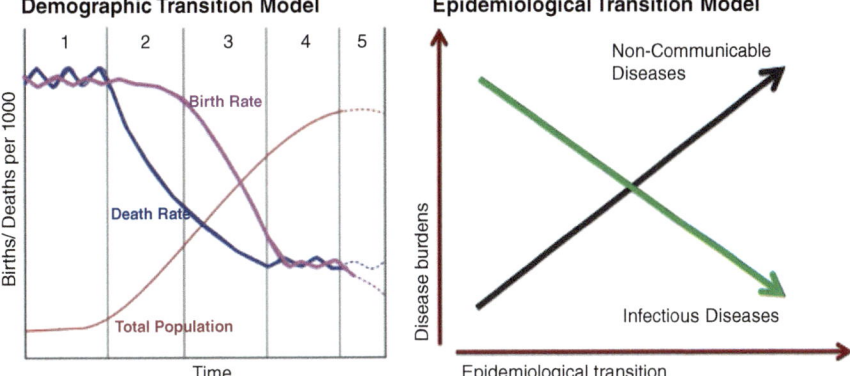

Fig. 5.4 Demographic transition model & Epidemiological transition model

5.7 How to Manage NCDs

Globally, NCDs only receive 1–2% of financing investment for health, despite causing 75% of deaths annually. Sustainable development goal (SDG) 3.4 aims to reduce the premature mortality from NCDs by one-third by 2030 [5]. The WHO has published The Global NCD Compact, in order to try and accelerate progress on prevention and control [6]. It focuses on the following five areas:

- saving, by 2030, the lives of 50 million people from dying prematurely of NCDs by implementing the most *cost-effective measures to prevent and control* NCDs;
- protecting 1.7 billion people living with NCDs by ensuring that they have *access to the medicines* and care they need during *humanitarian emergencies;*
- integrating NCDs within primary health care and *universal health coverage*;
- comprehensive *NCD surveillance and monitoring*; and,
- meaningfully engaging 1.7 billion people living with NCDs and mental health conditions in *policy-making and programming* [6].

The WHO has recommended NCD 'Best Buys', which are evidence-based, cost effective public health measures to help prevent and control NCDs. They include some of the following (list not extensive):

Tobacco
- Increase taxes and prices on tobacco products
- Comprehensive bans on tobacco advertising
- Eliminate exposure to second-hand tobacco smoke in all indoor workplaces, public places, public transport

Alcohol
- Increase taxes on alcoholic beverages
- Restrictions on exposure to alcohol advertising (across multiple types of media)
- Enact and enforce restrictions on the sale of alcohol

Unhealthy Diet
- Reformulation policies for healthier food and beverage products (e.g. reduction of saturated fats, free sugars and/or sodium)
- Comprehensive food labelling on packages
- Policies to protect children from the harmful impact of food marketing on diet

Physical Inactivity
- Campaigns to promote physical activity

References

1. Non communicable diseases. Available from: https://www.who.int/news-room/fact-sheets/detail/noncommunicable-diseases
2. Dattani S, Spooner F, Ritchie H, Roser M. Causes of death. Our World in Data [Internet] 2023 Sep 22; Available from: https://ourworldindata.org/causes-of-death
3. The state of diabetes treatment coverage in 55 low-income and middle-income countries: a cross-sectional study of nationally representative, individual-level data in 680 102 adults – the Lancet Healthy Longevity. Available from: https://www.thelancet.com/journals/lanhl/article/PIIS2666-7568(21)00089-1/fulltext
4. Omran AR. The epidemiologic transition: a theory of the epidemiology of population change. Milbank Q. 2005;83(4):731–57.
5. SDG Target 3.4 Non-communicable diseases and mental health. Available from: https://www.who.int/data/gho/data/themes/topics/sdg-target-3_4-noncommunicable-diseases-and-mental-health
6. Global NCD compact 2020-2030. Available from: https://www.who.int/initiatives/global-noncommunicable-diseases-compact-2020-2030

Chapter 6
Infectious Diseases – The Big Three

Hannah Raval

6.1 Introduction

Infectious diseases, also known as communicable diseases, are those that can be transmitted from person to person either directly or indirectly. Pathogenic microorganisms such as fungi, viruses, parasites or bacteria are the cause of these diseases, which can be spread through contact with bodily fluids, insect bites or through the air. Previously, communicable diseases were the biggest killer worldwide; however, due to d*emographic and epidemiological changes*, they no longer feature in the top 10 causes of death globally [1]. This being said, communicable diseases still account for 6 out of the top 10 causes of death and disability in low-income countries and marginalised populations [2].

In this chapter, we are going to focus on the 'Big Three'—HIV/AIDS, tuberculosis (TB) and malaria. HIV remains a major global public health issue, and 1.5 million people die each year from TB. In addition, nearly half of the world's population is at risk of malaria, and it is one of the biggest killers of children under 5 [3]. In 2002, an organisation called The Global Fund charity was set up to specifically address these three infectious diseases. In the past 20 years, the Global Fund partnership has invested more than US $60 billion, reducing the death rate caused by these three diseases by more than half [4]. However, they are still within the top 10 causes of death in low-income countries, alongside diarrheal disease, lower respiratory infections and a significant cause for neonatal deaths.

Despite a shift in focus in recent years towards non-communicable diseases, Sustainable Development Gaol 3.3 still aims 'by 2030, [to] end the epidemics of AIDS, tuberculosis, malaria and neglected tropical diseases and combat hepatitis, water-borne diseases and other communicable diseases' [5]. As well as deaths,

H. Raval (✉)
School of Medicine, Cardiff University, Cardiff, UK
e-mail: hannah.raval@doctors.org.uk

© The Author(s), under exclusive license to Springer Nature
Switzerland AG 2024
A. Fiander, G. Fry (eds.), *A Healthcare Students Introduction to Global Health*,
https://doi.org/10.1007/978-3-031-66563-9_6

43

communicable diseases can pose a major international health security threat, as seen during the COVID-19 pandemic. During this time, we were all affected by the truly global nature of infectious diseases, and therefore, communicable diseases remain a major challenge within field of Global Health.

We recognise there are many more infectious diseases that have a significant impact globally. Of note, respiratory infections, hepatitis and sexually transmitted infections cause a major burden. In Tropical Medicine, parasitology and a group known as 'Neglected Tropical Diseases' (NTDs) also play a major role. As this textbook aims to provide an overview, we will only be discussing the 'Big Three' in this chapter.

6.2 HIV/AIDS

6.2.1 Background

The Human Immunodeficiency Virus (HIV) originates from the simian immunodeficiency virus affecting chimpanzees. It is thought that it first spread to humans through bush meat hunting and coming into contact with affected animal's blood. By the mid-80s, the HIV pandemic had spread across the world [6]. AIDS (acquired immunodeficiency syndrome) was first recognised in 1981 when increasing numbers of homosexual men were being affected by opportunistic infections and rare malignancies.

In low-income countries, over half of adults affected by HIV are women. Most of the transmission has occurred through heterosexual transmission, when a partner has an unknown HIV status. Despite recent advances in diagnosis and treatment, HIV is still a major global health concern. Since the first recorded case, HIV has taken 40.4 million lives, and there are currently an estimated 39 million people living with HIV, two-thirds whom are from Sub-Saharan Africa [7]. Despite there being no cure, improvements in prevention, diagnosis and treatment have allowed many people affected by HIV to live healthy lives. At the time of writing, 86% of people living with HIV know their status, and 71% have suppressed viral loads [7].

6.2.2 HIV Transmission

HIV is transmitted via bodily fluids such as blood, semen, vaginal secretions and breast milk. The probability of transmission increases with viral load. At-risk groups include men who have sex with men, intravenous drug users, healthcare workers and those who have unprotected sex. There is also a risk of vertical transmission from mother to child, which is highest during labour and breast feeding. However, it is important to note that people on treatment, with an undetectable viral load, are not able to transmit HIV to sexual partners.

6.2.3 HIV Lifecycle

HIV is a retrovirus that is able to integrate its DNA into the host genome, making it very difficult to eradicate. The HIV life cycle includes binding, fusion, reverse transcription, integration, replication, assembly and budding. Once in the host cell, viral RNA is transcribed into DNA and is integrated into the host cell DNA. It is then able to replicate using the host cell infrastructure, budding off to create more viruses. The retrovirus binds itself via the $CD4^+$ receptor, which are found on the surface of T helper cells. The infection and destruction of T cells and macrophages, which are an integral part of the body's immune system, eventually leads to their depletion, resulting in immunodeficiency (Fig. 6.1).

6.2.4 HIV Signs and Symptoms

Seroconversion occurs in the first few weeks after an infection with HIV, and people may present with a flu-like illness. Following this, there is usually an asymptomatic latent phase which may last for many years (WHO Stage 1). Over time, the immune system weakens, leading to weight loss and mild opportunistic infections (stage 2). This can worsen, causing fevers, swollen lymph nodes, diarrhoea and a cough may develop. At this point, people are more susceptible to severe and persistent infections (stage 3), in particular, tuberculosis (TB).

Stage 4 is the AIDS defining condition, which occurs when the CD4 T helper cell count is below <200 per μL. At this stage, the immune system is severely impaired, resulting in infections such as Pneumocystis jirovecii pneumonia (PCP), cryptococcal meningitis, severe bacterial infections and cancers such as lymphomas and Kaposi's sarcoma.

Without treatment, people are expected to live between 9 and 11 years with the disease. As with many conditions, the earlier it is detected, the better the outcome for the patient. If the diagnosis is left until the onset of AIDS-associated symptoms, patients often only live for 6–19 months more. The leading causes of death with HIV are TB, especially in sub-Saharan Africa, then closely followed by Hepatitis C (Fig. 6.2).

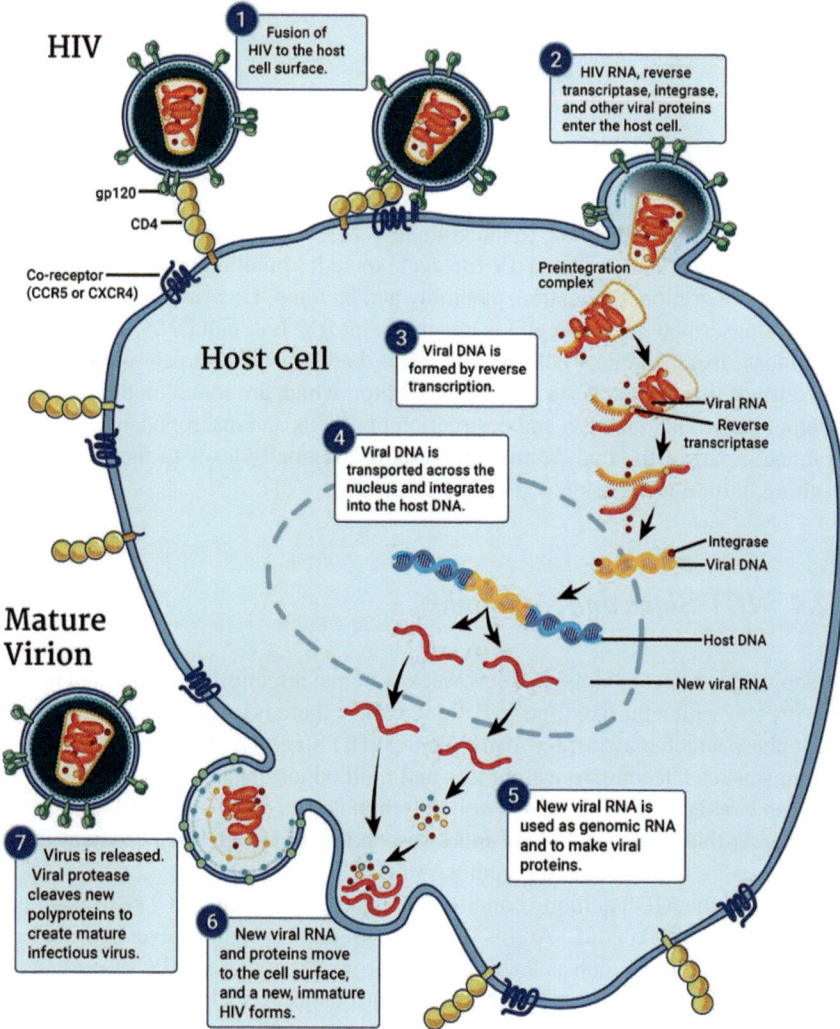

Fig. 6.1 HIV replication cycle [8]

6.2.5 *Diagnosis of HIV*

Rapid diagnostic tests are commonly used in high prevalence settings. Alternatively, fourth-generation ELISA tests can detect antibodies and p24 antigens within 14 days of exposure to the virus.

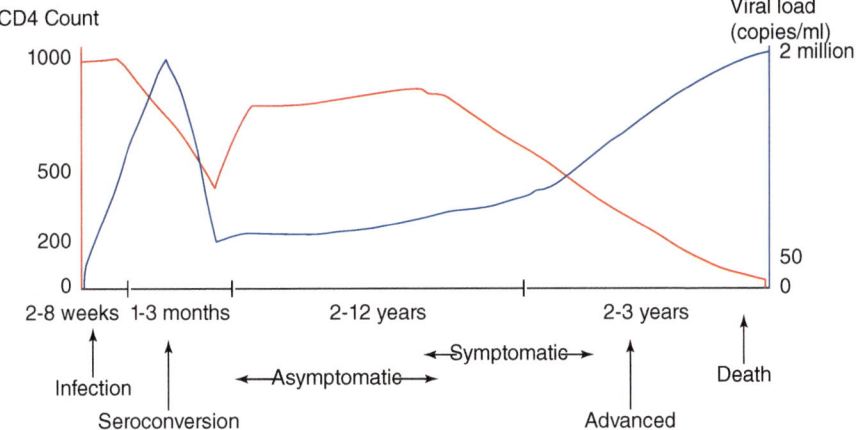

Fig. 6.2 Typical course of HIV infection if left untreated

6.2.6 Treatment

There is no cure for HIV; however, antiretroviral therapy (ART) taken lifelong can suppress the viral load to such an extent that the individual can live a long and healthy life. There are many different treatment regimens, with the most being common triple therapy including a combination of Tenofovir, Lamivudine and Dolutegravir. Treatment failure remains a significant issue, often secondary to poor adherence, poor absorption, inappropriate dosing or drug interaction. In high-income countries, genotypic testing can help tailor treatment regimens; however, in most low-income settings, treatment is tailed based on local protocols.

For many years, the expense and resources required for antiretroviral treatments limited and focused HIV management to cheap, preventative methods such as condoms and education of the general public. However, at the turn of the millennium, after much lobbying and pressure from charitable groups, manufacturers began to make more affordable ARTs. With the rollout of ARTs in South Africa, which is one of the countries with the highest HIV prevalence, the decline in HIV-associated mortality has resulted in an increase in the national life expectancy from 54 to 65 over the last 10 years [9].

6.2.7 Prevention of HIV

HIV is a preventable disease. The risks of transmission can be reduced through use of condoms, regular STI testing, voluntary male circumcision and safe needle exchange programmes. Medical treatment such as pre-exposure prophylaxis (PrEP) can also reduce the risk for vulnerable groups.

Through education regarding the importance of treatment adherence, the viral load can be adequately suppressed such that the viral load is <40 copies/mL. Undetectable viral load = untransmissible [10].

6.3 Tuberculosis

6.3.1 Background

TB is a chronic bacterial infection caused by the *mycobacterium tuberculosis* complex. It is spread through inhalation of infectious droplets, which can survive for a significant time in the environment. Most people will breathe in these droplets without contracting TB; however, it may cause disease in those who are immunocompromised. Roughly 25% of the global population have been infected with latent TB; however, only 5–10% of those infected will develop the disease.

Tuberculosis (TB) is the second leading cause of death due to an infectious disease worldwide. In 2020, ten million people contracted TB, and there were 1.5 million TB-related deaths [11]. The End TB strategy is a WHO initiative that works globally, aiming to reduce TB-related deaths by 95% by 2035 [12].

6.3.2 Presentation of TB

There are two stages to untreated tuberculosis:

- *Primary infection:* This is when TB is first inhaled into the lungs. The primary infection is usually asymptomatic or mild. Granulomas form to contain the bacterium. These can then either calcify, eliminating the disease or the bacterium can remain dormant within the granuloma, causing latent infection.
- *Secondary infection:* This is a reactivation of dormant TB granulomas when an individual becomes immunosuppressed. Immunosuppression can be induced through pregnancy, HIV or AIDS, malnutrition, diabetes or tobacco smoking. The reactivation can occur anywhere in the body: pleura, meninges, lymphatic system, blood, bones and joint (particularly of the spine).

Most TB cases have an insidious onset, and therefore, patients often present late with secondary infections. TB should be considered when at-risk groups are presenting with malaise, weight loss and night sweats. There may be organ-specific symptoms, depending on where reactivation occurs. In pulmonary TB, it is common to have a productive cough with blood stained sputum.

Due to their immunocompromised status, TB–HIV co-infection is extremely common, with TB being the leading cause of death in people living with HIV.

6.3.3   Diagnosing TB

Diagnosis is through the use of rapid molecular diagnostic tests, in particular Gene Xpert analysis of sputum samples. Other tests involve sputum microscopy, X-ray and the tuberculin skin test. Rapid tests are becoming more widespread; however, diagnosing multi-drug-resistant TB is still a challenge.

6.3.4   Treatment of TB

TB can be cured with a 6-month course of four antibiotics: rifampicin, isoniazid, ethambutol and pyrazinamide. It is important that patients have good adherence and complete the full course, in order to prevent drug resistance developing. Multi-drug-resistant TB (MDR-TB) is that which does not respond to two of the first-line antibiotics. The most common causes of this are inappropriate use of TB treatment and poor-quality drugs. These patients must then be treated with second-line antibiotics. These drugs are more cytotoxic, have longer drug courses, are more expensive and are not always available.

6.3.5   Prevention of TB

TB prevention includes education regarding the disease and droplet spread. Managing the environment is beneficial, such as ensuring adequate ventilation and good hygiene, such as covering your mouth when coughing. Early detection and case finding can help ensure timely treatment.

The BCG vaccine is a live vaccine that is given to people at risk and is most effective at preventing severe disease in children. In the UK, it is given to infants from high-risk families and to health workers. It is one of the most widespread vaccines worldwide and has been given to 80% of infants in countries where it is part of the childhood immunisation programme. It protects against disseminated TB; however, it does not protect against primary disease or prevent against reactivation of a latent pulmonary infection.

6.4 Malaria

6.4.1 Background

Malaria was originally named in Italy by physicians who believed the disease to be caused by dirty air—'mal aria'. In 1880, however, Charles Louis Alphonse Laveran identified the malaria parasite in the blood of one of his patients, a discovery that eventually led to him being awarded the Nobel Prize. Malaria is a disease spread to humans by infected *Anopheles* mosquitos, which carry the parasite from the Plasmodium group. The parasite travels through the human blood stream and leads to high fevers, and in some cases, can result in death. The WHO estimates around 560,000 people died in 2019 from malaria, most of whom were children [12].

There are five different species, all of the *Plasmodium* genus, that are capable of causing malaria in humans. They are found in different places across the world and have different incubation times. They are, however, almost exclusively confined to the tropics, as the following map depicts (Fig. 6.3).

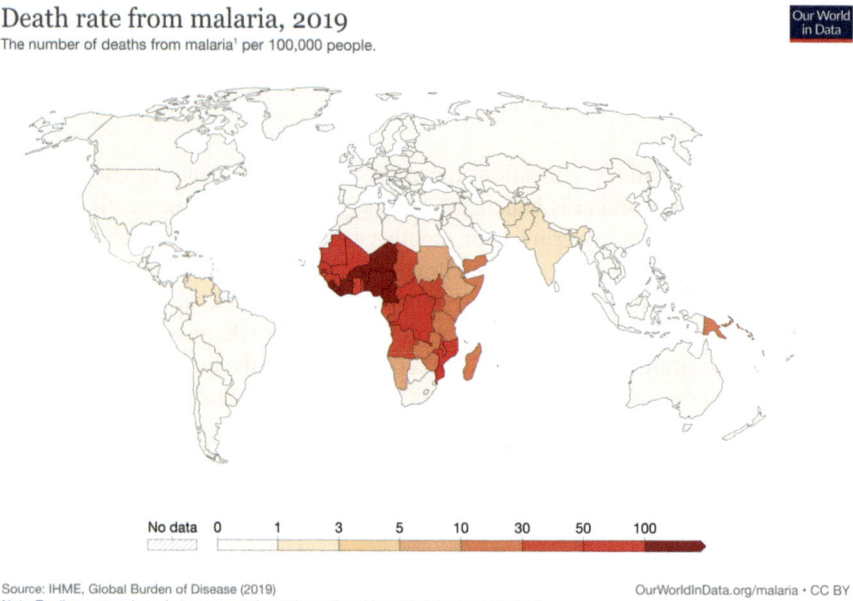

Death rate from malaria, 2019
The number of deaths from malaria¹ per 100,000 people.

No data 0   1   3   5   10   30   50   100

Source: IHME, Global Burden of Disease (2019) OurWorldInData.org/malaria · CC BY
Note: To allow comparisons between countries and over time this metric is age-standardized.

1. **Malaria**: Malaria is a life-threatening disease caused by parasites that are transmitted by female Anopheles mosquitoes. There are five parasite species that cause malaria in humans. Two of these species – P. falciparum and P. vivax – pose the greatest threat. The first symptoms – fever, headache and chills – usually appear 10 to 15 days after the infective mosquito bite and may be mild and difficult to recognize as malaria. Left untreated, P. falciparum malaria can progress to severe illness and death within 24 hours.

Fig. 6.3 Shows the global incidence of malaria worldwide in 2019 [13]

6.4.2 Malaria Parasite Life Cycle

The two most common species of malaria are *Plasmodium falciparum,* mostly found in Africa, and *Plasmodium vivax*, which is more common in South East Asia. All five species are transmitted between individuals by the female *Anopheles* mosquito, which acts as a vector and is unaffected by the parasite itself. The *Anopheles* mosquito breeds in water sources and is a night time biter. It feeds every 3 days.

Malaria life cycle [14].

1. The mosquito bites one human and draws some blood that is infected with the malaria parasite into its stomach.
2. The parasite in the form of Gametocytes then sexually reproduces to form Sporozoites, which can travel to the salivary glands of the mosquito after 10–18 days.
3. When the insect takes its next meal from an uninfected human, it injects its saliva (which has anticoagulant properties) into the subject's bloodstream, which includes the parasite in the form of Sporozoites.
4. The Sporozoites travel in the saliva into the host's bloodstream and to the host liver, where they mature into Schizonts within the liver cells. This stage produces no symptoms. Some species of *Plasmodium* can also stay dormant in the liver, leading to disease relapse in future years.
5. Symptoms only occur once the Schizonts rupture and enter the blood circulation in the form of Merozoites. This stage is known as the erythrocytic phase.
6. Merozoites are capable of infecting more red blood cells, where they undergo further multiplication, creating more Merozoites to infect more red blood cells, continuing the cycle of infection and eruption, which is what causes the cyclical fevers.
7. Some Merozoites differentiate into sexual forms called Gametocytes.
8. When the human host is bitten by another *Anopheles* mosquito, these Gametocytes are ingested and the lifecycle within the mosquito starts again. The full cycle takes 14 days (Fig. 6.4).

6.4.3 Clinical Presentation of Malaria

The symptoms of malaria are very non-specific and often present like a flu-like illness. Adults living in areas with high levels of malaria may build immunity and are often asymptomatic. The first symptoms usually develop 10–15 days after being bitten by an infected mosquito. Therefore, it is an important condition to remember in a 'returning traveller' who presents with a fever.

Symptoms
• Febrile illness—fevers every 48–72 hours
• Headache

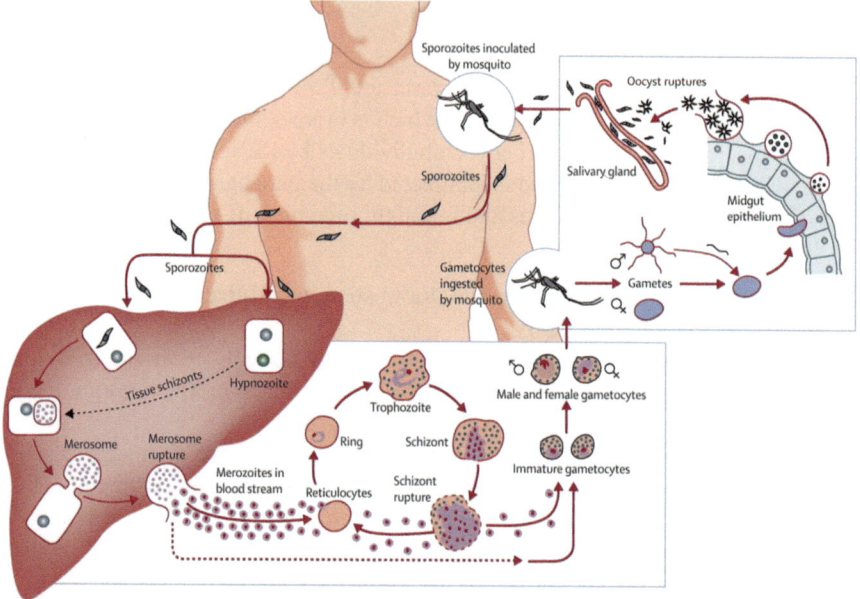

Fig. 6.4 Complex life cycle of the human malaria parasite *Plasmodium vivax* [15]

- Tiredness
- Cough
- Myalgia
- Abdominal pain
- Diarrhoea and vomiting

Signs
- Rigors
- Hepatosplenomegaly
- Jaundice
- Anaemia

The prognosis of the disease largely depends on the patient's immune status and the type of malaria that they have contracted. People who are immunocompromised, extremes of age or those who have never been exposed to the disease before are most likely to die of malaria. The signs of severe life-threatening malaria include bleeding, acidosis, hypoglycaemia, severe anaemia and renal failure. Another complication is cerebral malaria, which is more common in children, resulting in impaired consciousness, seizures and death. Life-threatening malaria is most often seen following infection with the *Plasmodium falciparum* species.

6.4.4   Diagnosing Malaria

Malaria is often diagnosed clinically; however, there are many tests available. The gold standard is through Blood Smear Microscopy, looking at thick and thin blood films. Most commonly, it is diagnosed using Rapid Diagnostic Tests (RDTs), which are cheap and easy to use. They are fast and sensitive; however, they are not able to differentiate between different species. Other methods include PCR analysis.

6.4.5   Treatment of Malaria

Due to growing drug resistance, malaria should always be treated with a variety of medications. Most commonly, uncomplicated malaria is treated with a 3-day course of Artemisinin Combination Therapy (ACT). This kills the parasite in all stages and prevents onwards transmission. The exact drug regimen will vary in different areas according to variables such as the species of Plasmodium parasite and local patterns of drug resistance. For severe malaria, intravenous Artesunate is used. Many anti-malarial drugs can have unpleasant neurological and psychiatric side effects.

6.4.6   Prevention of Malaria

Due to the method of transmission of the disease, measures for the prevention of malaria largely involve vector control. This includes bite prevention, such as wearing long clothes and using insecticides. More long-lasting methods include the implementation of mosquito nets that are sprayed with insecticides and indoor residual DDT spraying in malaria-ridden areas. Another method is through source reduction, by removing stagnant water where mosquitoes breed and chemical larvicide in breeding grounds.

Current research is exploring the genetic manipulation of the *Anopheles* mosquitoes so that they will be unable to transmit the malaria parasite in the future. Since 2021, the WHO is recommending the use of the RTS,S malaria vaccine among children in areas with a high *P. falciparum* transmission rate [16].

For people travelling to malaria affected areas, chemoprophylaxis is recommended. There are various regimens that include daily medication, such as Doxycycline or Malerone, all with their own side-effect profile.

6.4.7   WHO Action Plan for Malaria

The WHO finalised a Global Technical Strategy for Malaria in 2015 which is aimed to be met by 2030 [17]. This action plan aims to:

1. reduce malaria mortality and incidence rates globally.
2. eliminate malaria completely from at least 35 countries.
3. prevent the re-establishment of malaria in all countries that have been deemed malaria-free.

References

1. Bigna JJ, Noubiap JJ. The rising burden of non-communicable diseases in sub-Saharan Africa. Lancet Glob Health. 2019;7(10):e1295–6.
2. The top 10 causes of death [Internet]. [cited 2023 Sep 26]. Available from: https://www.who.int/news-room/fact-sheets/detail/the-top-10-causes-of-death
3. Our work: communicable and non-communicable diseases, and mental health [Internet]. [cited 2023 Sep 26]. Available from: https://www.who.int/our-work/communicable-and-noncommunicable-diseases-and-mental-health
4. About the Global Fund [Internet]. [cited 2023 Sep 26]. Available from: https://www.theglobalfund.org/en/about-the-global-fund/
5. SDG Target 3.3 Communicable diseases [Internet]. [cited 2023 Sep 26]. Available from: https://www.who.int/data/gho/data/themes/topics/sdg-target-3_3-communicable-diseases
6. Merson MH, O'Malley J, Serwadda D, Apisuk C. The history and challenge of HIV prevention. Lancet. 2008;372(9637):475–88.
7. HIV and AIDS [Internet]. [cited 2023 Sep 26]. Available from: https://www.who.int/news-room/fact-sheets/detail/hiv-aids
8. HIV Replication Cycle | NIH: National Institute of Allergy and Infectious Diseases [Internet]. 2018 [cited 2023 Nov 28]. Available from: https://www.niaid.nih.gov/diseases-conditions/hiv-replication-cycle
9. Doan T, Shin W, Mehta N. To what extent were life expectancy gains in South Africa attributable to declines in HIV/AIDS mortality from 2006 to 2017? A life table analysis of age-specific mortality. Demogr Res. 2022;46:547–64.
10. HIV Undetectable=Untransmittable (U=U), or Treatment as Prevention | NIH: National Institute of Allergy and Infectious Diseases [Internet]. 2019 [cited 2023 Sep 26]. Available from: https://www.niaid.nih.gov/diseases-conditions/treatment-prevention
11. Tuberculosis (TB) [Internet]. [cited 2023 Sep 26]. Available from: https://www.who.int/news-room/fact-sheets/detail/tuberculosis
12. The end TB strategy [Internet]. [cited 2023 Sep 26]. Available from: https://www.who.int/publications-detail-redirect/WHO-HTM-TB-2015.19
13. Roser M, Ritchie H. Malaria. Our World in Data [Internet]. 2019 Nov 12 [cited 2023 Sep 26]; Available from: https://ourworldindata.org/malaria
14. CDC – DPDx – Malaria [Internet]. 2020 [cited 2023 Sep 26]. Available from: https://www.cdc.gov/dpdx/malaria/index.html
15. Mueller I, Galinski MR, Baird JK, Carlton JM, Kochar DK, Alonso PL, et al. Key gaps in the knowledge of Plasmodium vivax, a neglected human malaria parasite. Lancet Infect Dis. 2009;9(9):555–66.

16. WHO recommends groundbreaking malaria vaccine for children at risk [Internet]. [cited 2023 Sep 26]. Available from: https://www.who.int/news/item/06-10-2021-who-recommends-groundbreaking-malaria-vaccine-for-children-at-risk
17. World Health Organization. Global technical strategy for malaria 2016–2030 [Internet]. Geneva: World Health Organization; 2015. [cited 2023 Sep 26]. 29 p. Available from: https://iris.who.int/handle/10665/176712

Chapter 7
Neglected Tropical Disease (NTDs)

Stephen Bates, Jonathan Peirce, and Anna Biju

7.1 Introduction

The definition of neglected tropical disease (NTD) has evolved over time from its initial conception; however now, the consensus is that NTDs are considered a diverse group of neglected endemic tropical diseases that primarily impact poor and marginalised populations [1].

The World Health Organisation (WHO) has set out a definitive list of 20 NTDs that require particular attention in the coming decade:

List of NTDs (as defined by WHO)			
Buruli ulcer	Chagas disease	Dengue and chikungunya	Dracunculiasis
Echinococcosis	Food-borne trematodiasis	Human African trypanosomiasis	Leishmaniasis
Leprosy	Lymphatic filariasis	Mycetoma, chromoblastomycosis and other deep mycoses	Onchocerciasis
Rabies	Scabies and other ectoparasitoses	Schistosomiasis	Soil-transmitted helminthiases
Snakebite envenoming	Saeniasis and cysticercosis	Trachoma	Yaws

The term was first introduced by the WHO to call for the spotlight to be focused on these previously overlooked diseases.

S. Bates (✉) · J. Peirce · A. Biju
School of Medicine, Cardiff University, Cardiff, UK
e-mail: batessp@cardiff.ac.uk; Anna.Biju3@wales.nhs.uk

© The Author(s), under exclusive license to Springer Nature Switzerland AG 2024
A. Fiander, G. Fry (eds.), *A Healthcare Students Introduction to Global Health*,
https://doi.org/10.1007/978-3-031-66563-9_7

7.2   Case Study 1: Dengue

7.2.1   *Introduction*

Dengue is a viral infection caused by four serologically different types of dengue virus (DENV 1–4) [2]. Dengue is an arbovirus, meaning it is spread by insects. These viruses, all members of the *Flaviviridae* family, have rapidly spread throughout the tropical and subtropical regions over the past 50+ years and continue to persist through their primary vector, the *Aedes aegypti* mosquito [2]. In recent years, there has been debate as to whether dengue is deserving of NTD classification as it is more generally recognised than other NTDs. On the other hand, as with the other NTDs, dengue lacks the sufficient spending and interventions at a community level, justifying its NTD classification [3].

- Patients with dengue fever classically present with a high fever of 40 °C lasting just under a week as well as a combination of the following signs and symptoms [2] (Fig. 7.1):
- lethargy,

Fig. 7.1 Macular rash in dengue [4]

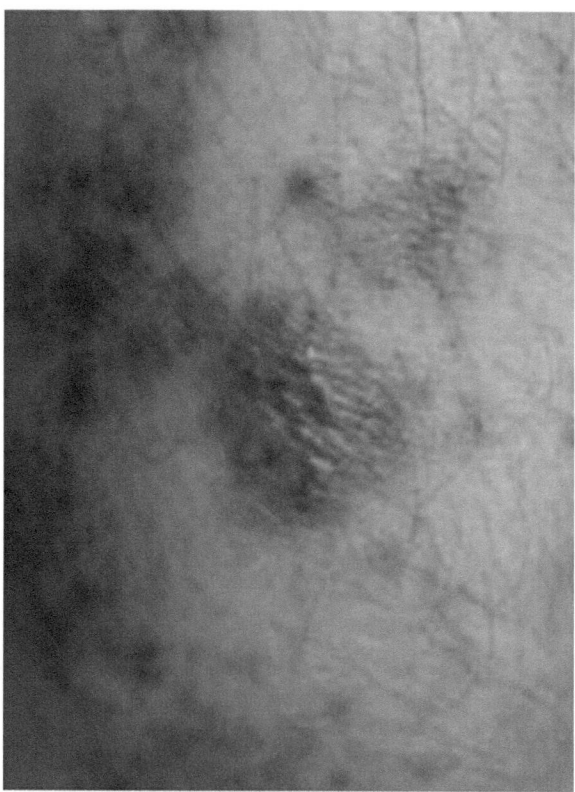

- headache,
- vomiting,
- myalgia,
- arthralgia,
- macular rashes.

In severe cases, dengue can develop into dengue haemorrhagic fever (DHF) and dengue shock syndrome (DSS). DHF usually occurs in children, although it can also occur in adults [5]. Dengue fever typically presents with 2 to 7 days of fever [6]. As this fever drops, this is when DHF may occur [5]. It frequently presents with skin haemorrhages and less commonly with epistaxis and bleeding gums as well as haemorrhage in other sites [6]. Because of plasma leakage [5], the patient can become shocked, which is described as dengue shock syndrome (DSS). The increase in plasma permeability that causes DHF and DSS frequently recovers in 2–3 days; in the meantime, the patient must be supported with aggressive fluid replacement therapy and close monitoring [6].

Dengue is notoriously difficult to diagnose in its initial stages without laboratory testing due to its different clinical presentations. In addition to this, infection with one viral serotype does not guarantee lifelong immunity. It is possible to become re-infected with the other viral serotypes [7, 8].

7.2.2 Burden of Disease

Dengue infects approximately 400 million people every year; however, this figure is likely to be higher since many cases are not formally diagnosed. Seventy-five per cent of those infected with dengue are asymptomatic and therefore go unreported. Dengue causes 10,000–50,000 deaths a year and was responsible for just under three million DALYs in 2017 alone.

Nearly 50% of the world's population in over 128 countries are at risk of contracting dengue as shown in the map below. There are even some areas where all four serotypes of the virus are present (Fig. 7.2).

7.2.3 How Is Dengue Currently Managed?

Currently, there is no specific treatment for dengue aside from supportive care. Fluid replacement therapy and paracetamol as an analgesic and antipyretic are the mainstay of management [10].

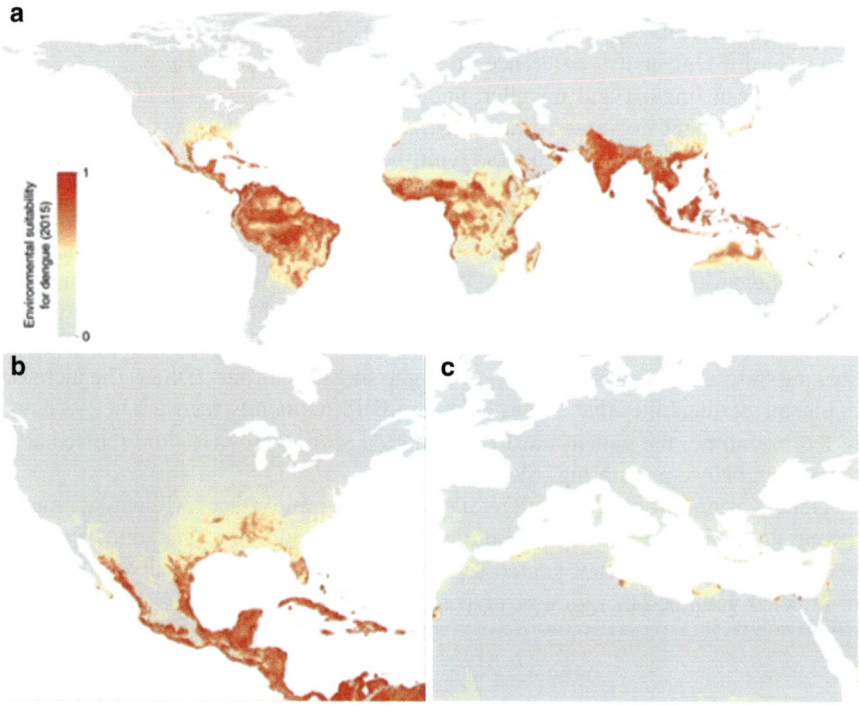

Fig. 7.2 Countries 2015 probability of dengue [9]

7.2.4 What Are the Solutions to Dengue?

7.2.4.1 Vector Control

Without a specific treatment, limiting the burden of this disease is dependent on stringent prevention methods such as vector control [1]. This can be achieved by:

1. Removing stagnant water sources and covering water tanks with lids which can serve as breeding grounds for mosquitos.
2. Utilising nets, coils, repellents, and appropriate clothing to prevent mosquito bites during the day as well as to prevent mosquito entry into homes.

7.2.4.2 Disease Surveillance

Significant disease surveillance allows governments to identify outbreaks of the disease early and promptly implement the relevant prevention methods. This can be complemented by the education of communities in dengue endemic nations on the symptoms of dengue and easy prevention methods [1].

7.2.4.3 Vaccination

Vaccine development for dengue is ongoing; one vaccine has already been approved for use with moderate success in individuals who have had a previous dengue virus infection. However, as of yet, there is no vaccination for individuals who have no history of dengue infection.

7.3 Case Study 2: Leprosy

7.3.1 Overview

Leprosy, also known as Hansen's disease, is caused by *Mycobacterium leprae*. It is an NTD that is passed on via droplet transmission. The disease is characterised by at least one of three signs in the clinical setting including hypopigmented or erythematous skin patches with loss of sensation, thickening of peripheral nerves and the detection of acid-fast bacilli on relevant smears or biopsies. Schwann cells of peripheral nerves are infected by *M. Leprae* leading to the nerve damage and subsequent disabilities [11]. If left untreated, leprosy can have lifelong effects such as severe physical disability, besides subsequent social issues for the individual [12]. Leprosy is treatable with multidrug therapy consisting of the antimicrobials dapsone, clofazimine and rifampicin (Fig. 7.3).

7.3.2 Burden of Disease

In 2019, a total of 119 countries reported new cases of leprosy with 80% of the burden concentrated in India, Brazil and Indonesia. Furthermore, 82 out of 119 countries reported new cases with Grade 2 Disabilities (G2D) which represents visual deformities. The WHO classifies the physical disabilities of leprosy with reference to three categories (Fig. 7.4):

Grade of disability	Definition
Grade 0	Absence of disability (including no anaesthesia) and absence of visible damage or deformities on eyes, hands and feet
Grade 1	Loss of protective sensibility in the eyes, hands or feet, without visible damage or deformities
Grade 2	Presence of deformities or visible damage to the eyes, hands or feet

Fig. 7.3 'Typical lesions' of leprosy seen as erythematous patches on the skin [13]

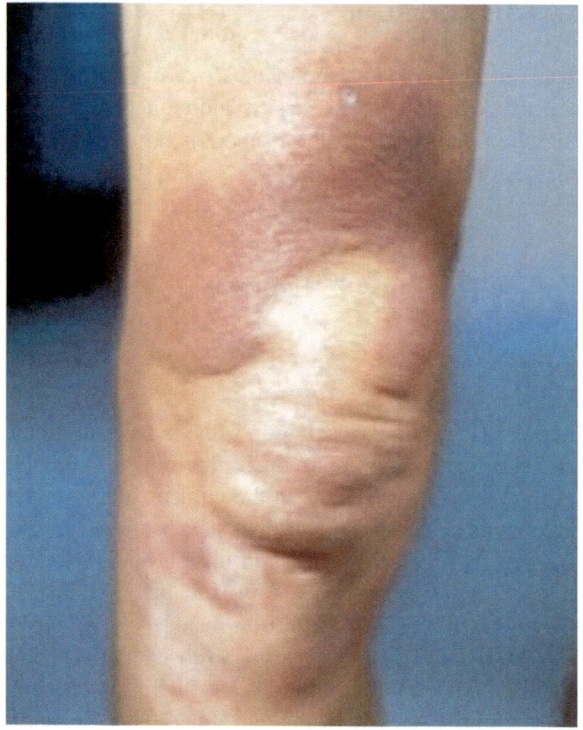

7.3.3   Social Stigma

Historically, individuals with leprosy have been subject to discrimination and marginalisation from society on account of their condition. In some cases, leprosy can cause significant physical disfigurement, and individuals express being viewed with a sense of 'fear and loathing' as a result. In extreme cases, this rejection from society even extends to denial of water access. This social isolation has a well-recognised effect on the mental health of those with the condition and can deter them from presenting to the healthcare services.

7.3.4   Current Progress

The WHO *Global Leprosy Strategy 2016–2020* document placed global targets to achieve by 2020 which were centred on reducing paediatric cases and new G2D cases to highlight the need for early detection and treatment as well as to ensure a reduction in transmission. Additionally, reducing discrimination and its effects against people with leprosy has been included within the targets.

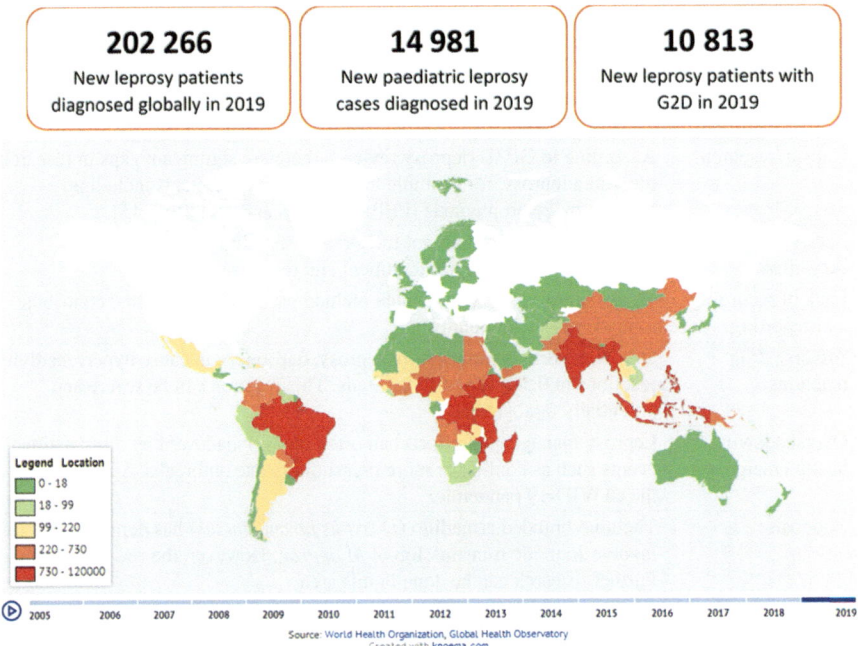

Fig. 7.4 World map showing the number of new cases reported in 2019 [12]

Impact indicator	2020 target	2019 status
G2D rate in newly detected cases	< 1/million population	1.4/million population
Newly detected child cases with G2D	Zero	Reported: 370 Estimated: 400–500
Number of laws allowing discrimination on the basis of leprosy	Zero countries with discriminatory laws	127 discriminatory laws in 22 countries

7.3.5 The Main Challenges of Leprosy Management in LRCs (Based on those Identified by World Health Organisation, 2021)

Detection delay	May be due to insufficient diagnostic capacity, poor contact tracing programmes, lack of symptom awareness in communities and leprosy-associated stigma (can avoid self-reporting)
Limited skills, resources, and access	Lack of political interest and inadequate funding may explain the limited clinical skills and resources available (including laboratory services). Additionally, limited access and referral to services—for example surgery, self-care training, physical rehabilitation and psychological support services

Stigma and discrimination	As explored previously, in some countries, patients with leprosy are often victims of discrimination and can even be denied basic human rights—previously established leprosy awareness programmes on improving leprosy-based knowledge have not illustrated any significant improvements in this area [14]
Gaps in research	According to GPZL (leprosy review), there are significant gaps in research regarding leprosy, for example in diagnostics, treatments including post-exposure prophylaxis (PEP), vaccines and disability [15]
Lack of routine surveillance	Surveillance systems are not fully established in most countries thus reducing chances of early treatment and reducing spread
Lack of recording and reporting	Weak recording systems (which include paper-based systems) contribute to inadequate data quality
Adverse drug reactions	One of the drug treatments for leprosy, dapsone, can cause hypersensitivity reactions in 0.5–3.6% of individuals. This reaction can be severe and potentially fatal [16]
Overshadowing health emergencies	Leprosy management efforts can often be overshadowed by other national events such as conflict or more pressing disease outbreaks. As seen with the COVID-19 pandemic.
Zoonosis	The nine-branded armadillo (*Dasypus novemcinctus*) has demonstrated to involve zoonotic transmission of *M. leprae*. However, the risk is low. Further research can be done in this area
Migration	Leprosy can be spread to previously uninfected countries by migration

7.3.6 Summary of Future Targets and Strategies

The 'Long-Term Vision' posed by the World Health Organisation (WHO) aims for:

Zero leprosy: zero infection and disease, zero disability, zero stigma and discrimination.

The global targets set in place to achieve by 2030: [17]
1. Zero reports of new endemic cases in 120 countries
2. Reduce the annual number of new cases detected by 70%*
3. Reduce annual rate per million population of new cases with G2D by 90%*
4. Reduce the rate per million children of new child cases with leprosy by 90%*
* From 2020 projected baseline

• *The Pillars of Strategy:* [17]

1. Establish zero-leprosy road maps in all endemic countries tailored to the nation
2. Boost leprosy prevention and integrated active case detection

3. Additional focus on management of leprosy and its complications whilst preventing new disabilities
4. Ensure all human rights are respected and eliminate stigma

7.4 Case Study 3: Trachoma

Trachoma is caused by recurrent infection of the conjunctiva by the bacteria *Chlamydia trachomatis*. Chronic infection can lead to visual impairment or blindness. It is the leading infectious cause of blindness in the world [18]. Trachoma is a disease of poverty, overcrowding and poor sanitation [19]. It can be treated with antibiotics and surgery [18].

7.4.1 World Health Organisation Statistics on the Burden of Trachoma

Trachoma is a public health problem in 44 countries and is responsible for the blindness or visual impairment of about 1.9 million people. A total of 137 million people live in trachoma endemic areas and are at risk of blindness as a result [1].

7.4.2 Trachoma and Visual Impairment (Fig. 7.5)

A simplified grading system can be used to understand how trachoma can lead to visual impairment [20]. There are six stages:

1. *Normal conjunctiva*—the normal conjunctiva is pink, smooth and thin.
2. *Follicular (FH) trachomatous inflammation*—the conjunctiva becomes red and inflamed; at this stage, fewer than five conjunctival follicles (round collections of lymphocytes) can be seen.
3. *Intense (TI) trachomatous inflammation*—the conjunctiva becomes intensely inflamed, and more than five follicles can be identified.
4. *Trachomatous scarring (TS)*—inflammation leads to scarring on the conjunctiva.
5. *Trachomatous trichiasis (TT)*—a scarred conjunctiva turns inwards such that the eyelashes contact the eye.
6. *Corneal opacity (CO)*—abrasion of the cornea leads to opacity which can cause a person to become visually impaired or blind.

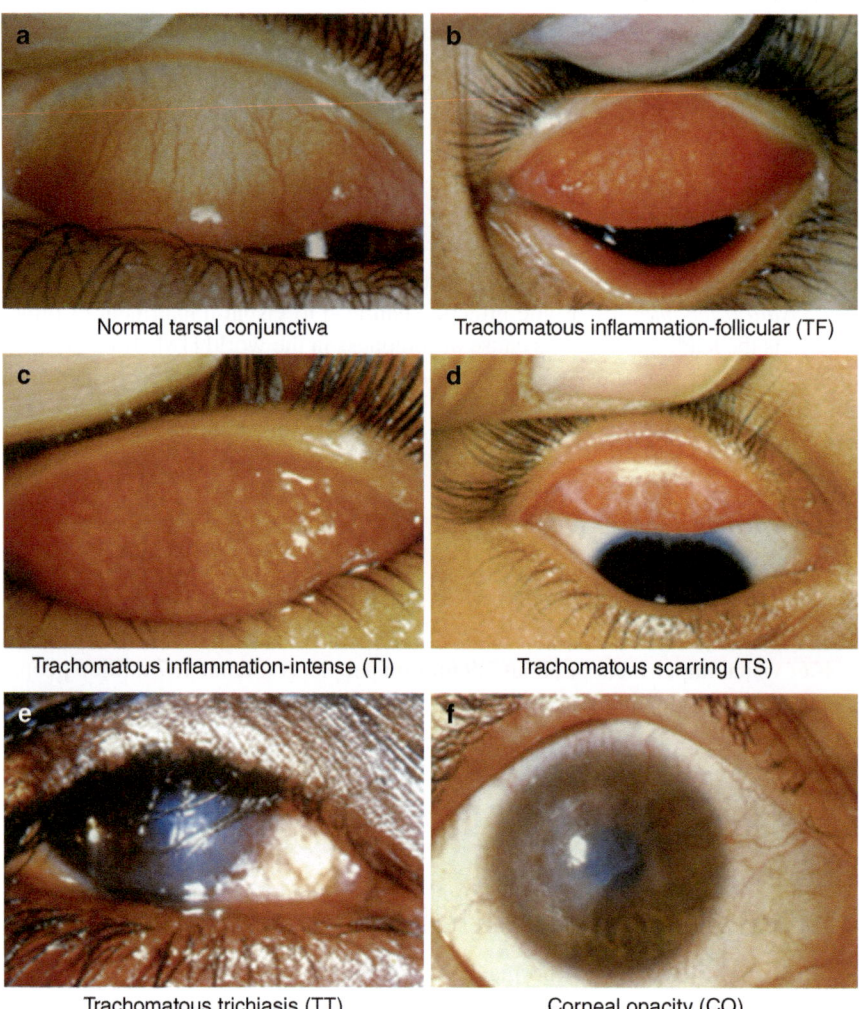

Fig. 7.5 The stages of trachoma [20]

7.4.3 Example Case Study (Fig. 7.6)

Haimamote Debebe is a woman living in a remote area of Ethiopia. Together with her husband, they keep livestock.

Two years ago, she began to experience crippling pain in her eyes as well as headaches. Her sight has deteriorated such that she cannot recognise faces, look after the livestock or take care of herself. A local eye care worker diagnosed her with trachoma, but she is unsure whether she will be able to access the antibiotics and surgery needed to treat the condition.

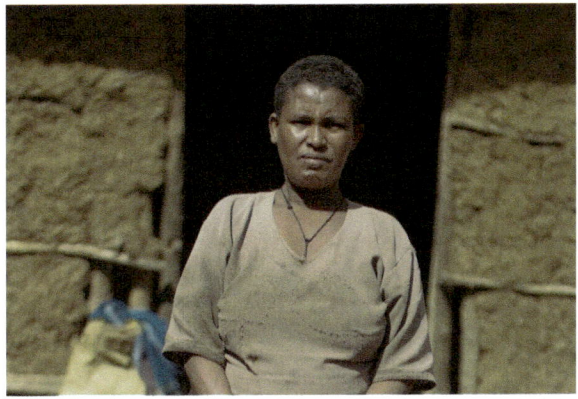

Fig. 7.6 Haimamote Debebe lives in a remote area of Ethiopia and suffers with trachoma [21]

Women account for 80% of the disability-adjusted life years (DALYs) linked to trachoma-related visual impairment [22]. It is thought that water-based domestic activities such as washing clothes, bathing young children and cooking increase the risk of contracting the infection [21].

7.4.4   Interventions to Reduce the Burden of Trachoma

The WHO has recently released a strategy for the elimination of trachoma entitled SAFE [23]. It has four elements:

1. *Surgery*—surgery is the most effective way of preventing a person from becoming blind due to trachoma, but there are still issues regarding access.
2. *Antibiotics*—great steps forward have been made in terms of access to antibiotics with the creation of single or few dose azithromycin.
3. *Facial cleanliness*—unless mass antibiotic administration is to be continued indefinitely, developments must be made in sanitation, and these have included campaigns on facial cleanliness.
4. *Environmental improvement*—improved latrines and water sanitation will act to reduce the prevalence of trachoma.

7.5   Summary

It is evident from the NTDs explored that they are fundamentally united by their impact on deprived nations. Common strategies for elimination encompass vector control, improved sanitation and education running alongside coordinated prevention programmes.

The WHO has set the following summative goals to promote the elimination of NTDS [1]:

- Decrease the number of people requiring treatment for NTDs by 90%
- Ensure the elimination of at least one NTD in 100 countries or more
- Eradicate dracunculiasis and yaws
- Reduce by 75% the disability-adjusted life years (DALYs) related to NTD

Thirty-three countries have eliminated at least one NTD since 2012 [21]. By implementing the people-centred approach as defined by the WHO, further progress towards the targets for 2030 can be achieved. However, action towards addressing NTDs is dependent on the political commitment of individual countries, and there remains much work to be done.

References

1. Ending the neglect to attain the Sustainable Development Goals: A road map for neglected tropical diseases 2021–2030: World Health Organisation; 2020 [cited 2023 1/10/2023]. Available from: https://www.who.int/publications/i/item/9789240010352.
2. Hasan S, Jamdar SF, Alalowi M, Al Ageel Al Beaiji SM. Dengue virus: a global human threat: review of literature. J Int Soc Prev Community Dent. 2016;6(1):1–6.
3. Horstick O, Tozan Y, Wilder-Smith A. Reviewing dengue: still a neglected tropical disease? PLoS Negl Trop Dis. 2015;9(4):e0003632.
4. Huang HW, Tseng HC, Lee CH, Chuang HY, Lin SH. Clinical significance of skin rash in dengue fever: a focus on discomfort, complications, and disease outcome. Asian Pac J Trop Med. 2016;9(7):713–8.
5. World Health O. Dengue haemorrhagic fever: diagnosis, treatment, prevention and control. 2nd ed. Geneva: World Health Organization; 1997.
6. Gubler DJ. Dengue and dengue hemorrhagic fever. Clin Microbiol Rev. 1998;11(3):480–96.
7. Beltrán-Silva SL, Chacón-Hernández SS, Moreno-Palacios E, Pereyra-Molina JÁ. Clinical and differential diagnosis: dengue, chikungunya and Zika. Revista Médica del Hospital General de México. 2018;81(3):146–53.
8. Aguas R, Dorigatti I, Coudeville L, Luxemburger C, Ferguson NM. Cross-serotype interactions and disease outcome prediction of dengue infections in Vietnam. Sci Rep. 2019;9(1):9395.
9. Messina JP, Brady OJ, Golding N, Kraemer MUG, Wint GRW, Ray SE, et al. The current and future global distribution and population at risk of dengue. Nat Microbiol. 2019;4(9):1508–15.
10. Guzman MG, Gubler DJ, Izquierdo A, Martinez E, Halstead SB. Dengue Infect Nat Rev Dis Primers. 2016;2:16055.
11. Bhat RM, Prakash C. Leprosy: an overview of pathophysiology. Interdiscip Perspect Infect Dis. 2012;2012:181089.
12. Integrating neglected tropical diseases in global health and development: World Health Organisation; 2019 [cited 2021 1/10/2021]. Available from: https://www.who.int/neglected_diseases/resources/9789241565448/en/.
13. Ramos-e-Silva M, Rebello PFB. Leprosy. Am J Clin Dermatol. 2001;2(4):203–11.
14. Mankar MJ, Joshi SM, Velankar DH, Mhatre RK, Nalgundwar AN. A comparative study of the quality of life, knowledge, attitude and belief about leprosy disease among leprosy patients and community members in Shantivan leprosy rehabilitation Centre, Nere, Maharashtra, India. J Glob Infect Dis. 2011;3(4):378–82.

15. Steinmann P, Dusenbury C, Addiss D, Mirza F, Smith WCS. A comprehensive research agenda for zero leprosy. Infect Dis Poverty. 2020;9(1):156.
16. Liu H, Wang Z, Bao F, Wang C, Sun L, Zhang H, et al. Evaluation of prospective HLA-B*13:01 screening to prevent Dapsone hypersensitivity syndrome in patients with leprosy. JAMA Dermatol. 2019;155(6):666–72.
17. Towards zero leprosy. Global leprosy (Hansen's Disease) strategy 2021–2030: World Health Organisation; 2021 [cited 2023 1/10/2023]. Available from: https://www.who.int/publications/i/item/9789290228509.
18. Lansingh VC. Trachoma. BMJ Clin Evid. 2016;2016:0706. PMID: 26860629; PMCID: PMC4748511
19. Stocks ME, Ogden S, Haddad D, Addiss DG, McGuire C, Freeman MC. Effect of water, sanitation, and hygiene on the prevention of trachoma: a systematic review and meta-analysis. PLoS Med. 2014;11(2):e1001605.
20. Thylefors B, Dawson CR, Jones BR, West SK, Taylor HR. A simple system for the assessment of trachoma and its complications. Bull World Health Organ. 1987;65(4):477–83.
21. Living With Trachoma: Uniting To Combat NTDs; 2023 [updated May 2019; cited 2023 01/10/2023]. Available from: https://unitingtocombatntds.org/en/neglected-tropical-diseases/resources/living-with-trachoma/.
22. Burton MJ, Mabey DC. The global burden of trachoma: a review. PLoS Negl Trop Dis. 2009;3(10):e460.
23. Bailey R, Lietman T. The SAFE strategy for the elimination of trachoma by 2020: will it work? Bull World Health Organ. 2001;79(3):233–6.

Chapter 8
Sexual Health in Low- and Middle-Income Countries (LMICs)

Sarah Morgan, Samuel Kelland, and Alice Cassie

> **Definition**
> Sexual health, as with health in general, is not just the absence of disease but
> '...*a state of physical, emotional, mental and social well-being in relation to*
> *sexuality*' [1].

8.1 What Makes Good Sexual Healthcare?

Key elements of good sexual healthcare include:

- A respectful, open and positive approach.
- Understanding sexual health with regards to social, political and cultural aspects within a community.
- Involving all age and genders, including the young and elderly.
- Ensuring wide accessibility.
- Acceptance of diverse forms of sexuality and its expression.
- Fulfilling basic human rights in regard to sexual health.

However, good sexual health provision has several barriers which prevent it from being globally accessible. Some occur to an extent all over the world, and others are more problematic in low resource countries.

S. Morgan (✉) · S. Kelland · A. Cassie
School of Medicine, Cardiff University, Cardiff, UK
e-mail: sarahcmorgan@doctors.org.uk; Alice.Cassie@nhs.net

A. Fiander, G. Fry (eds.), *A Healthcare Students Introduction to Global Health*,
https://doi.org/10.1007/978-3-031-66563-9_8

8.2 Barriers to Sexual Health Coverage

8.2.1 Social, Religious and Cultural Beliefs within a Community

1. *Gender Inequalities*

    Gender inequalities often arise in relation to perceived gender norms and societal expectations. Gender stereotypes can be especially harmful in relation to sexual and reproductive health. For example, women in certain cultures may be expected to be more passive and submissive to males in the family. This prejudice then translates to less independence and control over sexual health decisions such as contraception or condom use.

2. *Social taboos*

    In many cultures and societies, sex and sexuality can be taboo subjects. This makes open and honest conversation difficult and limits the impact of sexual health education. The taboo nature of the topic can also lead to prejudices and stigmatisation against certain groups going unchallenged and proliferating, for example, against homosexual and transgender communities.

3. *Religious/Cultural beliefs*

    Certain practices and beliefs may oppose advances in sexual and reproductive health. Opposition to contraception and condoms in a community can make prevention of sexually transmitted infections (STI) and unwanted pregnancy difficult. It can also cause problems with funding and provision through certain charities. This is seen with some conservative Christian charities refusing to fund health services that advocate or provide condoms.

8.2.2 Political, Economic and Structural Factors

4. *Political*

    Whilst international bodies such as the World Health Organisation and United Nations have promoted and set targets for widening access to sexual health, this is not always necessarily followed on a national level. Different governments often fail to prioritise the rollout of comprehensive sexual health services.

5. *Economic*

    Funding and financial planning for sexual health can be limited, particularly in low resource countries. This issue can be compounded if the political structures and governments have little political will to change the situation.

6. *Structural and geographic factors*

    In many countries, populations in rural areas find it difficult to access sexual health services due to factors such as long distances and poor infrastructure for transport.

8.3   Sexual Health Conditions in LMICs

Certain sexual health conditions are overlooked in LMICs due to failed prioritisation or lack of resources. The list of conditions is extensive; however, here we use STIs and cervical cancer as examples.

8.3.1   Sexually Transmitted Infections (Other than HIV)

- STIs are a preventable and easily treated area of sexual health; however, they are often not well provided for in low resource countries.
- Annually, an estimated 200 million women are infected with either chlamydia, gonorrhoea, syphilis or trichomoniasis. Yet, an estimated 8 in 10 women of these women receive no medical treatment [2]. Diagnosed and treated in their early stages, all four of these common STIs can be treated with antibiotics with no long-term consequences.
- However, screening in low resource countries is poor. This can be related back to the diagnostic tests being relatively expensive and needing lab facilities and trained staff which are often unavailable.

> STI prevention and early treatment could prevent further complications such as pelvic inflammatory disease, infertility or the transmission of syphilis to newborns.

8.3.2   Cervical Cancer

Human papillomavirus (HPV) is a common STI which is thought to affect almost every sexually active individual at some point in their lifetime. For most, there will be no consequences; however, in rare cases, certain high-risk HPV types may cause cervical cancer.

Cervical cancer is the second most common cancer amongst females, affecting an estimated 530,000 women a year [3]. The vast majority of cervical cancer deaths occur in LRCs. This is because of poor prevention and late detection. Cervical screening utilises either cytology or HPV testing of exfoliated cervical cells, undertaken at intervals for women over a certain age. Abnormal cells that have the potential to become cancerous are identified and monitored or treated to prevent progression.

8.4 Prevention

Gardasil 9 is currently being used in vaccination programmes. This vaccine protects against HPV strains 6, 11, 16, 18, 31, 33, 45, 52 and 58.

- HPV strains 6 and 11 are associated with genital warts. Whilst HPV strains 16, 18, 31, 33, 45, 52 and 58 increase the risk of cervical cancer. [4]
- These vaccines, given to 12–13-year old girls and boys in the UK, are thought to decrease long-term rates of cervical cancer; however, cost is still a major barrier to implementation in many areas.
- Another area of research is to make cheaper methods of detection, and one possibility is inspection by eye with acetic acid (visual inspection with acetic acid or VIA), where a trained professional can identify pre-invasive abnormalities.

8.5 What Role Does Contraception, Abortion and the Management and Prevention of STIs Have in Promoting Sexual Health?

For over 40 years, the importance of contraception, safe abortion and the prevention of STIs has been at the centre of international policies for promoting sexual health. This was re-emphasised in the United Nations (UN) Sustainable Development Goals (SDG) [5].

8.5.1 Contraception and Abortion

The use of contraception has increased globally to an approximate 874 million women using a form of modern contraception. Yet despite this, 164 million women had an unmet contraceptive need in 2022, whereby they wanted to either delay or avoid pregnancy but were not using contraception [6]. Annually, around 121 million unintended pregnancies occur with up to 61% of unintended pregnancies globally ending in abortion in both countries with legal and restricted abortion access.

Unsafe abortions are defined by the WHO as 'a procedure for terminating an unintended pregnancy either by persons lacking the necessary skills or in an environment lacking the minimal medical standards, or both' [7].

Due to these unwanted pregnancies, it is estimated that around 20 million women undergo unsafe abortions every year, with this practice contributing to 13% of maternal deaths worldwide [8]. Therefore, it has been recognised as an important issue in achieving the SDG for reducing the maternal mortality ratio.

The following are the factors listed by the WHO that influence the incidence of unwanted pregnancies and unsafe abortions:

- Access of young women and young men to information on contraception.
- The legality of supplying contraceptives to unmarried young people.
- The legality of abortion.
- Sociocultural norms and practices regarding sex outside marriage.
- Unintended pregnancies and the provision of safe abortion.
- The influence of gender-power relations on the ability of girls and women to use contraceptive methods, or to reject sexual relations with men.
- The readiness of the health service to provide safe abortions to the full extent of the law.

Making abortion safe for women is a priority due to its contribution to maternal mortality, but this needs to be achieved alongside reduction in the number of unwanted pregnancies.

8.6 Contraception and STIs

Barrier contraception plays a dual role in preventing pregnancy as well as preventing STI transmission. One million people acquire a new STI infection every day, [9] highlighting the scale of the problem.

Access to contraception has once again been highlighted as an area that needs to be improved to reduce STI transmission rates, especially in the lower- and middle-income countries where there is a relative high burden of sexually transmitted infections [10]. This method relies heavily on having easy access for communities to contraception, but also the knowledge on how to use it effectively.

The use of condoms as a barrier form of contraception is an essential element in preventing STIs and HIV, even if they are not the most effective method for preventing pregnancy [11]. Dual protection may be promoted: condoms to prevent STI and a more highly effective method of contraception, e.g. LARCs, to prevent pregnancy.

Education of adolescents and young men and women has been a focus of many initiatives to promote sexual health in LMICs. But research shows that education alone is not enough and must be complemented with economic, cultural and geographic access to reproductive sexual health [12].

This is essential as STI infections, alongside their immediate symptoms, can have a profound and lifelong effect on people's health. Potential morbidities include:

- Pregnancy complications
- Pelvic inflammatory disease
- Infertility
- Certain cancers, such as HPV-associated cervical and rectal cancer
- Arthritis
- Recurrent genital warts

8.7 Infertility and Sexual Health

8.7.1 Causes of Infertility

Across the world, infertility affects millions of individuals affecting up to one in six adults, with a broadly similar prevalence in high-income (17.8%) and LMICs countries (16.5%). The causes of infertility worldwide affect both men and women, and include structural abnormalities of the reproductive tract, hormonal and wider endocrine disorders as well as lifestyle and environmental factors. Some causes of infertility are considered more specific to LMICs.

Causes of infertility in LMICs include:

- Pelvic inflammatory disease (PID) which causes scarring of the fallopian tubes. It is caused by STIs such as chlamydia and gonorrhoea
- Genital tuberculosis (TB) which is common in areas with high TB prevalence
- Post-partum or post-abortal sepsis/infection
- Malaria
- Sickle cell disease
- Drinking water contaminated with arsenic or pesticides, causing infertility in men
- The practice of female genital mutilation (FGM)
- Consanguineous partnerships.

8.7.2 Cultural Implications of Infertility

There is a social stigma associated with infertility, with high levels of distress reported by individuals that may lead to infertility-related stress, depression and anxiety. Whilst both male and female factors may be the cause of infertility, women often perceive and experience higher levels of stigma, shame and negative psychological effects [13]. Different spiritual, religious and cultural backgrounds can affect understanding and beliefs surrounding infertility and shape how it affects relationships in families and communities.

8.7.3 Managing Infertility in LMICs Countries

Fertility treatments such as in vitro fertilisation (IVF) come at a huge cost to both individuals and healthcare systems [14]. Therefore, prevention has typically been a focus of fertility treatment in low-middle income countries. Methods of infertility prevention include education regarding contraception, especially barrier methods and dual protection, and the long-term complications of untreated STIs and therefore the importance diagnosis and early treatment of infection.

Whilst prevention of infertility has been key, a focus in more recent years has included the spread of affordable infertility treatment including assisted reproductive technologies (ARTS), which include more invasive treatments such as IVF. There remain significant barriers in terms of economic viability, as well as varied cultural preconceptions and associated stigma [15].

8.8 Gender-Based Violence and Sexual Health

Gender-based violence (GBV) is….

- *Any violence that occurs because of perceived gender roles*
- *Unequal power relationships between men and women in society*
- *Violence including physical, mental or sexual harm or suffering as well as coercion, threats and deprivation of liberty* [16]

Traditional gender-based roles within cultures and societies have an impact on gender-based violence. Although a global issue and affecting all demographics to some extent, the highest lifetime prevalence is for women in the 'least developed countries' according to most recent WHO data on gender-based violence [17].

8.8.1 The Importance of Tackling GBV

More than one-third of women will experience GBV at some point in their lives. GBV is inextricably linked with poorer overall health and has far-reaching sexual, psychological, social and physical implications [18].

Rape and violence are associated with increased risk of STI transmission and unintentional pregnancy. Unintentional pregnancy in turn can be associated with abortion, which can be illegal and unsafe, and is associated with medical complications which may result in death. Rape can also cause loss of status in a community and cause social isolation as a woman; this is especially rife during times of conflict when women are at increased risk of sexual violence [19].

How to tackle GBV…

- *Root causes*
  Often, cultural beliefs about women's role and low status in society create a culture of male dominance and sexual entitlement. By promoting gender equity in all walks of life, we can begin to close the gender power gap and in turn reduce GBV.
- *Risk factors*
  Substance abuse and depression are risk factors for perpetrating GBV; by treating these conditions, we decrease this risk.

- *Education*

  Most perpetrators of sexual crime begin to enact this behaviour in adolescence; by educating people from a young age, we can begin to prevent GBV and improve people's sexual health. When children are raised by parents who are equals and respect one another, they will learn 'good' behaviours for their own future relationships. Adverse childhood experiences (ACE) increase the risk of GBV.
- *Empowerment*

  By educating women, we are empowering them. This begins to change the role of women in society. Once they know about their rights, they can access services which will advocate for them, and help to keep them safe from violence.

References

1. World Health Organisation (2006) Defining sexual health, sexual health. Available at: http://www.who.int/reproductivehealth/topics/sexual_health/sh_definitions/en/
2. Sherris J. Cervical cancer in the developing world. West J Med. 2001;175(4):231–3. https://doi.org/10.1136/ewjm.175.4.231.
3. Cervical cancer statistics I world cancer research fund international [Internet]. 2022. Available from: https://www.wcrf.org/cancer-trends/cervical-cancer-statistics/
4. Burd EM. Human papillomavirus and cervical cancer. Clin Microbiol Rev. 2003;16(1):1–17. https://doi.org/10.1128/cmr.16.1.1-17.2003.
5. Department of Economic and Social Affairs. The 17 goals I sustainable development [Internet]. United Nations; [cited 2023 July 13]. Available from: https://sdgs.un.org/goals
6. United Nations Department of Economic and Social Affairs, Population Division. World Family Planning 2022: Meeting the changing needs for family planning: contraceptive use by age and method. UN DESA/POP/2022/TR/NO. 4. 2022. Available at: https://desapublications.un.org/publications/world-family-planning-2022-meeting-changing-needs-family-planning-contraceptive-use
7. Perveen S. The danger of unsafe abortions: Their causes and complications [Internet]. [cited 2023 July 13]. Available from: https://blogs.jpmsonline.com/2017/03/10/the-danger-of-unsafe-abortions-their-causes-and-complications/
8. Berer M. Making abortions safe: a matter of good public health policy and practice. Reprod Health Matters. 2002;10(19):31–44. https://doi.org/10.1016/s0968-8080(02)00021-6.
9. Sexually transmitted infections Factsheet (STIs). World Health Organization; 2022. Available at: https://www.who.int/news-room/fact-sheets/detail/sexually-transmitted-infections-(stis). Accessed 16 July 2023.
10. Mayaud P. Approaches to the control of sexually transmitted infections in developing countries: old problems and modern challenges. Sex Transm Infect. 2004;80(3):174–82. https://doi.org/10.1136/sti.2002.004101.
11. How effective is contraception at preventing pregnancy? [Internet]. NHS; 2020 [cited 2023 July 16]. Available from: https://www.nhs.uk/conditions/contraception/how-effective-contraception/
12. Desrosiers A, Betancourt T, Kergoat Y, Servilli C, Say L, Kobeissi L. A systematic review of sexual and reproductive health interventions for young people in humanitarian and lower-

and-middle-income country settings. BMC Public Health. 2020;20(1) https://doi.org/10.1186/s12889-020-08818-y.

13. Xie Y, Ren Y, Niu C, Zheng Y, Yu P, Li L. The impact of stigma on mental health and quality of life of infertile women: a systematic review. Front Psychol. 2023:13. https://doi.org/10.3389/fpsyg.2022.1093459.

14. Njagi P, Groot W, Arsenijevic J, Dyer S, Mburu G, Kiarie J. Financial costs of assisted reproductive technology for patients in low- and middle-income countries: a systematic review. Human Reprod Open. 2023;2023(2) https://doi.org/10.1093/hropen/hoad007.

15. Ombelet W. Global access to infertility care in developing countries: a case of human rights, equity and social justice. Facts Views Vision ObGyn. 2011;3(4):257–66.

16. U.N. declaration on the elimination of violence against Women. Enduring Violence. 2019;vii–viii. https://doi.org/10.1525/9780520948419-001.

17. Violence against women prevalence estimates, 2018: global, regional and national prevalence estimates for intimate partner violence against women and global and regional prevalence estimates for non-partner sexual violence against women. Geneva: World Health Organization; 2021.

18. WorldBank. Violence against women and girls—what the data tell us [Internet]. [cited 2023 July 16]. Available from: https://genderdata.worldbank.org/data-stories/overview-of-gender-based-violence/

19. Gender-based violence in emergencies [Internet]. 2023 [cited 2023 July 16]. Available from: https://www.unicef.org/protection/gender-based-violence-in-emergencies

Recommended Reading Resources: STI, Abortion and Contraception

20. Bearak J, Popinchalk A, Ganatra B, Moller A-B, Tunçalp Ö, Beavin C, et al. Unintended pregnancy and abortion by income, region, and the legal status of abortion: Estimates from a comprehensive model for 1990–2019. Lancet Global Health. 2020;8(9) https://doi.org/10.1016/s2214-109x(20)30315-6.

21. Global health sector strategies on, respectively, HIV, viral hepatitis and sexually transmitted infections for the period 2022–2030. Geneva: World Health Organization; 2022.

22. Haakenstad A, Angelino O, Irvine CM, Bhutta ZA, Bienhoff K, Bintz C, et al. Measuring contraceptive method mix, prevalence, and demand satisfied by age and marital status in 204 countries and territories, 1970–2019: a systematic analysis for the global burden of disease study 2019. Lancet. 2022;400(10348):295–327. https://doi.org/10.1016/s0140-6736(22)00936-9.

23. Berer M. 'Making abortions safe: a matter of good public health policy and practice', Reproductive Health Matters, 10, pp. 31–44. Abortion. 2002;2017:431–44. https://doi.org/10.4324/9781315263502-25.

24. Sexually transmitted infections Factsheet (STIs) (2022) World Health Organization. Available at: https://www.who.int/news-room/fact-sheets/detail/sexually-transmitted-infections-(stis). Accessed 16 July 2023.

25. Sully EA, Biddlecom A, Darroch JE, Riley T, Ashford LS, Lince-Deroche N, et al. Adding it up: investing in sexual and reproductive health 2019. New York: Guttmacher Institute; 2014. Available at: https://www.guttmacher.org/sites/default/files/report_pdf/adding-it-up-investing-in-sexual-reproductive-health-2019.pdf

Recommended Reading: Sexual Health and Infertility

26. Infertility Factsheet [Internet]. World Health Organization; 2023 [cited 2023 July 16]. Available from: https://www.who.int/news-room/fact-sheets/detail/infertility
27. Inhorn MC, Patrizio P. Infertility around the globe: new thinking on gender, reproductive technologies and global movements in the 21st Century. Human Reprod Update. 2015;21(4):411–26. https://doi.org/10.1093/humupd/dmv016.
28. Ombelet W. Global access to infertility care in developing countries: a case of human rights, equity and social justice. Facts Views Vision in ObGyn. 2011;3(4):257–66.
29. Rutstein SO, Shah IH. Infecundity infertility and childlessness in developing countries. Geneva: World Health Organization; 2004.

Recommended Reading: Gender Based Violence (GBV)

30. Decker MR, Miller E, Illangasekare S, Silverman JG. Understanding gender-based violence perpetration to create a safer future for women and girls. Lancet Global Health. 2013;1(4) https://doi.org/10.1016/s2214-109x(13)70085-8.
31. Violence against women prevalence estimates, 2018: global, regional and national prevalence estimates for intimate partner violence against women and global and regional prevalence estimates for non-partner sexual violence against women. Geneva: World Health Organization; 2021.

Useful Resources

32. Data on population, gender equality and sexual and Reproductive Health [Internet]. [cited 2023 July 16]. Available from: https://www.unfpa.org/data
33. Global health observatory [Internet]. World Health Organization; [cited 2023 July 16]. Available from: https://www.who.int/data/gho

Chapter 9
Maternal Health in Low Resource Countries

Jasmine Kew, Rachel Price, and Sarah Roberts

9.1 Introduction: The Statistics

In the UK, pregnancy is commonly viewed as a time of joy, happiness and new life. However, for many women around the world, pregnancy and childbirth can be life-threatening events:

- In 2020, there were an estimated 287,000 maternal deaths worldwide. This equates to approximately 800 a day, or 1 maternal death every 90 seconds [1]. Ninety-five per cent of these deaths occurred in low-income countries, and it is predicted that most of these could have been prevented [1].
- Following on from the millennium development goals, the more recent 2015 sustainable development goals (SDGs) identify the importance of improving maternal health worldwide. For example, the ambitious SDG target 3.1 aims to 'reduce the global maternal mortality ratio to less than 70 per 100 000 live births' [2]. Despite this, although maternal mortality rates have decreased over the past 15 years, the progress has been slow, and many countries are nowhere near reaching their targets.
- The standard measurement of maternal health is the *maternal mortality rate*— the number of maternal deaths per 100,000 of *all* births.
- Another commonly used measurement of maternal health is the *maternal mortality ratio*. This refers to the number of maternal deaths occurring in a specific time period per 100,000 *live* births in the same period which may be a more useful measurement as it allows us to state the estimated risk of death in a single pregnancy [3]. Since 1990, the global maternal mortality ratio (MMR) has dropped by only 2.6% annually [4].

J. Kew · R. Price · S. Roberts (✉)
School of Medicine, Cardiff University, Cardiff, UK

© The Author(s), under exclusive license to Springer Nature Switzerland AG 2024
A. Fiander, G. Fry (eds.), *A Healthcare Students Introduction to Global Health*, https://doi.org/10.1007/978-3-031-66563-9_9

- Pregnancy-associated *morbidity* is also important to consider as many more women will endure pregnancy-related illness during pregnancy or after giving birth.

9.2 Where Do Women Die?

9.2.1 Maternal Health Morbidity Disproportionately Affects Low Resource Countries

Maternal morbidity is a worldwide issue; however, the impact and statistics regarding maternal mortality and maternal morbidity vary drastically from country to country (see Fig. 9.1).

It is recognised by the World Health Organisation that 95% of women who die in childbirth live in low or low-middle-income countries [1]. Further scrutiny of these worldwide figures for maternal mortality [1] reveals that 70% of maternal deaths occur in Sub-Saharan Africa, and a further 17% are attributable to Central and

Maternal mortality ratio, 2017

The number of women who die from pregnancy-related causes while pregnant or within 42 days of pregnancy termination per 100,000 live births.

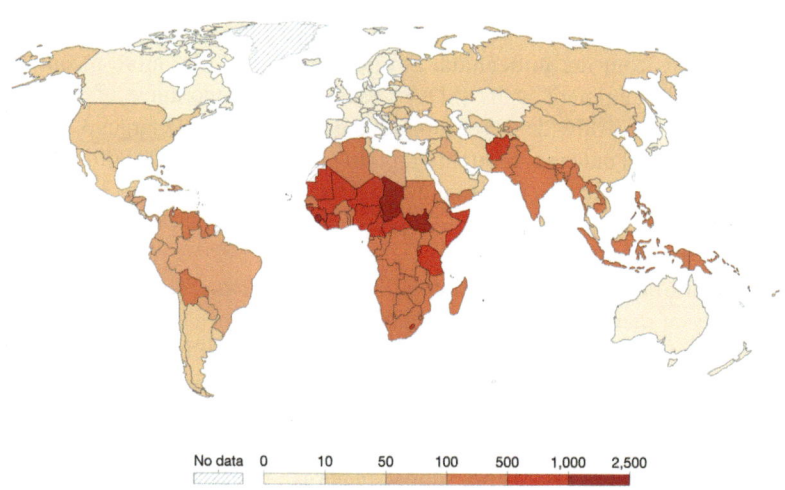

Fig. 9.1 Worldwide maternal mortality ratioThis shows a clear difference in maternal mortality between developed continents such as Europe and North America and developing countries including sub-Saharan Africa and parts of AsiaSource: MATERNAL MORTALITY RATIO (GAPMINDER (2010) AND WORLD BANK (2015)). Published online at OurWorldInData.org. Retrieved from https://ourworldindata.org/maternal-mortality#where-are-women-most-at-risk-of-dying-in-childbirth [5]

Southern Asia. By comparison, the risk of a woman dying due to maternal causes was 400 times lower in Australia or New Zealand than in Sub-Saharan Africa.

This data clearly shows a discrepancy between high- and low-income countries. It can therefore be suggested that maternal health statistics reflect the economic status of a country.

9.3 Causes of Maternal Mortality in Low-Income Countries

9.3.1 Medical Causes

Direct causes of maternal mortality account for 73% of reported deaths and relate to obstetric complications that occur during pregnancy, labour or in the first six weeks post delivery, or resulting from any medical treatment received [6]. Indirect deaths account for the remaining 27.5% and relate to pre-existing health conditions, which can be exacerbated by pregnancy, resulting in maternal death.

- *Haemorrhage*—blood loss that occurs before or during delivery accounts for a third of total deaths caused by haemorrhage, the remaining two-thirds occur after delivery, known as the postpartum phase [6]. Postpartum haemorrhage (PPH) can be minor, 500–1000 ml blood loss, or major >1000 ml lost, and classified as primary, or 'early', if blood loss is within 24 hours, and secondary, or 'late', if occurring more than 24 hours post delivery [7]. The most common cause is uterine atony, where the uterine muscle fails to contract leading to failure of occlusion of blood flow post delivery [8]. Other causes include:

  - Placental issues such as placenta previa, accreta and abruption.
  - Uterine rupture.
  - Trauma to the genital tract.
  - Retained placental tissue.
  - Maternal coagulation disorders.

- *Pre-eclampsia*—hypertensive disorders are the second leading cause of maternal deaths, the prevalence of which is highest in Latin America and Caribbean regions [6]. Pre-eclampsia was characterised by new onset of high blood pressure and protein in the urine, 'proteinuria', after 20 weeks' gestation, or in the postpartum period [9]. However, newer definitions describe it as a complex multisystem syndrome associated with new hypertension, and significant end-organ dysfunction (liver, kidney failure or central nervous system dysfunction) with or without proteinuria. The causes of pre-eclampsia are not fully understood but thought to be related to issues with the development of placental vasculature, leading to under perfusion and stress [10]. Risk factors include prior pregnancies with pre-eclampsia, diabetes, advanced maternal age and obesity. If pre-eclampsia is not diagnosed and treated, eclampsia and/or 'HELLP' can occur. Eclampsia refers to the presence of tonic-clonic seizures or coma in a patient with pre-eclampsia, in the absence of any other neurological condition. Patients can present with blurred vision, photophobia or confusion prior to developing seizures. *HELLP* syndrome is a triad of *H*aemolysis, *E*levated *L*iver enzymes and *Low P*latelets. It causes problems with blood clotting and can present with abdominal pain, nausea and vomiting. Mortality arises most often from massive stroke or liver rupture [11]. Foetal complications of pre-eclampsia include intrauterine growth restriction (IUGR), premature delivery and foetal death.

- *Infections & Sepsis*—obstetric infections are the third leading cause of maternal death, with most being 'maternal sepsis'; a life-threatening condition defined as organ dysfunction resulting from infection during pregnancy, childbirth, postabortion or the postpartum period [12]. Common infection sites include the urinary tract, the uterus 'endometritis', placenta and amniotic fluid 'chorioamnionitis', or skin/soft tissue involving postsurgical wound infections and mastitis. Postabortion-related infections also occur after direct trauma and injury to the uterus and vagina with foreign objects. Without timely treatment of these infections with antibiotics, sepsis can occur. Sepsis is defined as a 'life-threatening organ dysfunction caused by a dysregulated host response to an infection' [13]. In its most severe form known as 'septic shock', mortality rates are often over 40%. Signs and symptoms include fever, fast heart rate, increased work of breathing, low blood pressure, confusion or altered level of consciousness.
- *Delivery complications*—Obstructed labour or 'labour dystocia' occurs when the presenting part of the foetus cannot progress into the birth canal, despite strong uterine contractions [14]. It can arise due to a mismatch between foetal size and the mother's pelvis. The foetus may be larger in size due to gestational diabetes, or in areas of malnutrition, the pelvis of the mother may be smaller in size. Other causes include foetal malpresentation, where the foetus is not in the correct position for delivery. The only way to alleviate this is by means of a caesarean section, or by using instruments such as forceps or Ventouse, which may not be readily available in developing countries. Complications of an obstructed labour include infection, trauma to the genital tract, uterine rupture and haemorrhage. For the foetus, asphyxiation can occur leading to brain damage or death. A common and debilitating consequence of obstructed labour is the formation of an obstetric fistula—a hole which forms between the vaginal wall and the bladder and/or the rectal walls. Fistulas not only lead to further infections and complications, but also a host of social problems including divorce, exclusion from religious activities, separation from families, worsening poverty and extreme suffering by those women affected.
- *Unsafe abortion*—Around 45% of all abortions are 'unsafe', of which 97% take place in lower resourced countries [15]. It has been estimated that 7.9% maternal deaths occur due to unsafe abortion; however, this figure in reality is probably much higher due to underreporting and stigma [6]. Of the women that survive, many will suffer long-term health complications as a result. Methods of unsafe abortion include [16]:

  - Consuming toxic fluids—turpentine, bleach.

- Causing direct injury to the vagina and uterus—using foreign bodies, herbal preparations.
- Placing inappropriate medication into the vagina or rectum.
- External injury—falling from stairs, or roof, causing blunt trauma to abdomen.

The main causes of death from these practices include haemorrhage, infection and sepsis, genital trauma and bowel necrosis.

9.4 Social Barriers to Accessing Healthcare During Pregnancy and Labour

Antenatal care coverage is an indicator used to measure access to healthcare services during pregnancy. It is important as it represents both access to, and use of, maternity services [17]. Although the statistics vary dramatically from country to country, worldwide it is estimated that fewer than 65% of women see a skilled healthcare professional the recommended 4 times during pregnancy [18]. Complications that arise during pregnancy may therefore go undetected and untreated with potentially worse outcomes for both mother and child.

Factors that prevent women from seeking and/or receiving medical care during pregnancy are broad but include:

- *Financial Resources*—although in most areas of the UK maternal services are easily accessible and free at the point of use, this is often not the case in other countries where many women cannot afford to travel to and pay for medical attention. This is particularly a problem for antenatal services which are aimed at screening and health promotion, meaning that individuals often see little immediate benefit from utilising the service, and are thus reluctant to spend precious resources on care.
- *Distance to resources*—particularly within rural communities, hospitals and midwifery clinics can be great distances away from the population that they aim to serve. With poor road conditions, lack of transportation and lack of time and money for transportation, many women cannot easily get to official healthcare services to seek advice and medical care.
- *Lack of education and information* regarding maternal services—there is a relationship between lower levels of maternal education and higher maternal mortality. Reduced levels of education may lead to a lack of understanding of the importance of maternal care, in addition to a lack of knowledge regarding available services, thus reducing access to antenatal care and resulting in poorer maternal outcomes for this population.
- *Inadequate services*—worldwide there is a lack of trained healthcare workers in maternal health and accessible maternity services, with this shortage being particularly evident in less resourced nations. This may mean that even if women reach healthcare facilities, these are often poorly equipped to deal with obstetric

problems and are often oversubscribed with too few healthcare professionals and a lack of suitable equipment. Not only can this directly negatively affect maternal mortality and morbidity, it can perpetuate a lack of trust in the health service and contribute to reduced use of available services.

- *Cultural practices*—There is a host of evidence that has shown that even where healthcare services are available and accessible, many women still do not utilise them. Cultural traditions and beliefs vary enormously between communities within and across nations and can heavily influence an individual's decision to access healthcare and follow advice that may be given there. For example, a recent qualitative study examining the cultural barriers of accessing maternal healthcare in Pakistan identified that there was a tradition of 'wait and see' tactics even when obstetric complications were potentially lethal. Furthermore, it was the cultural norm in certain communities to require consent from the husband and/or mother-in-law to access a maternal healthcare professional and going out alone, even in an emergency, could bring great dishonour to the family [19].

9.5   What Interventions Have Been Introduced to Combat Maternal Mortality and How Effective Have these Interventions Been?

There are a multitude of specific medical interventions that can be implemented to prevent specific causes of maternal and neonatal mortality and morbidity [20], past the scope of this chapter. However, there are more general interventions that are also paramount.

9.5.1   Skilled Birth Assistants

- Having a skilled birth assistant (SBA) present at a birth helps improve outcomes for both mother and child. The SBA can be a doctor, nurse or midwife, trained specifically in maternal care. Their presence reduces mortality and morbidity as they identify warning signs of potential problems and act to mitigate these issues proactively.
- Sri Lanka, Malaysia and Honduras are countries that have managed to significantly reduce their MMRs between 1930 and 1995. This has been facilitated by increased political commitment and financial provision, resulting in the training of more SBAs and improved, more accessible maternity services [21].
- This being said, in the absence of universal commitment from all governments, financial strains, difficulty in recruiting and retaining SBAs, in addition to

logistical problems distributing SBAs to where they are needed, many women across the world still do not have access to, or seek, an SBA.

9.5.2   Providing Essential Medications

- Even when skilled birth assistants are available, lack of resources including medication may impede their ability to prevent or treat certain complications.
- Organisations such as Life for African Mothers [22] provide essential medications to treat birth complications. For example, magnesium sulphate for prevention of seizures in pre-eclampsia or treatment of seizures in eclampsia. Misoprostol is another low-cost and effective medication used to prevent and treat postpartum haemorrhage.
- Areas where these medications are readily available tend to have lower rates of maternal mortality than areas where these medications are in short supply.

9.5.3   Family Planning

- It is estimated that there are 220 million women of childbearing age who would like to delay or reduce childbearing but who are unable to access contraception [23].
- Access to a preferred method of contraception and family planning advice reduces the need for unsafe abortion and helps mothers limit the size of their families. Having fewer children enables parents to invest more time and finance into each child. A final advantage of family planning is that the use of barrier contraceptive methods prevents the transmission of sexually transmitted infections.

9.5.4   Abortion

- Where safe abortion is accessible and postabortion care is of a high standard, deaths from abortions are low [15].
- Shifting from surgical-based abortion to medical abortion could also help to improve access to safe abortions as more medical professionals can deliver safe medical abortion. This would also help to lower risks of surgery and anaesthesia-related complications and reduce costs to the healthcare system.

9.6   What Further Interventions Are Needed?

- Increased funding would help to improve access to essential drugs. Humanitarian organisations such as Life for African Mothers (https://www.lifeforafricanmothers.org) highlight the importance of funding for distributing misoprostol which is used in the management of postpartum haemorrhage. Improved logistical pathways and transport links would also help to improve the access and distribution of these medications.
- Working to improve communication between local healthcare providers and local hospitals could enable more women to receive timely and specialised medical attention and interventions when required. This would benefit from greater funding and expertise to improve these communication pathways.
- In addition, greater recruitment and training of skilled birth assistants in countries with a high MMR (such as Sub-Saharan Africa) would enable more women in these countries to access appropriate care during pregnancy and labour.
- Increased access to better family planning services could reduce the pressure on birthing facilities, meaning each individual birth can be more effectively managed.
- Widespread education about the danger signs for pregnant women can help reduce mortality, as the earlier potential problems are identified, the sooner and more successfully they can be treated. Detecting hypertension, proteinuria, STIs including HIV, anaemia and foetal malposition can all help to prevent maternal deaths.
- Decentralising care and providing care for women in their communities can mitigate transportation difficulties. This can also help women to access timely interventions such as caesarean section if required which can then help to reduce the risk of further complications such as the formation of obstetric fistulas. One example of this is the introduction of maternal waiting homes which have been shown to increase access and utilisation of maternity services [24].

9.7   Moving from Humanitarian Aid to Government Solutions

- Increased political commitment to reducing MMR results in better funding for maternal health, leading to improved healthcare facilities and more trained skilled birth assistants.
- In many lower resourced countries, there is a lack of political commitment to reducing national MMR. Therefore, international organisations and charities are largely responsible for interventions introduced to reduce maternal mortality. Arguably, this lack of governmental commitment is due to the low status of women in these countries, suggesting that a fundamental change in attitudes is

needed. Countries that have seen the most dramatic reductions in their MMR have been those with the most substantial governmental commitment.

References

1. World Health Organization. Maternal mortality key facts. In WHO; 2023 [cited 2023 June 12]. Available from: https://www.who.int/news-room/fact-sheets/detail/maternal-mortality
2. The Global Health Observatory, World Health Organization. SDG Target 3.1 Maternal mortality [Internet]. World Health Organization; [cited 2023 June 2]. Available from: https://www.who.int/data/gho/data/themes/topics/sdg-target-3-1-maternal-mortality
3. The Global Health Observatory, World Health Organization. Maternal Mortality Ratio [Internet]. World Health Organization; 2023 Jan [cited 2023 June 1]. Available from: https://www.who.int/data/gho/indicator-metadata-registry/imr-details/26#:~:text=Maternal%20mortality%20ratio%20%3D%20(Number%20of,household%20surveys%20or%20other%20sources
4. WHO, UNICEF, UNFPA, World Bank Group and UNDESA/Population Division. Trends in maternal mortality 2000 to 2020 Estimates by WHO, UNICEF, UNFPA, World Bank Group and UNDESA/Population Division [Internet]. Department of Sexual and Reproductive Health and Research World Health Organization; 2023 Feb [cited 2023 June 1]. Available from: https://data.unicef.org/resources/trends-in-maternal-mortality-2000-to-2020/
5. Roser M, Ritchie H. Maternal mortality. Our World in Data [Internet]. 2013.; Available from: https://ourworldindata.org/maternal-mortality
6. Say L, Chou D, Gemmill A, Tunçalp Ö, Moller AB, Daniels J, et al. Global causes of maternal death: a WHO systematic analysis. Lancet Glob Health. 2014 Jun;2(6):e323–33.
7. Prevention and Management of Postpartum Haemorrhage. Green-top Guideline No. 52. BJOG: Int Obstet Gy. 2017;124(5):e106–49.
8. World Health Organisation. WHO Recommendation on Tranexamic Acid for the Treatment of Postpartum Haemorrhage. [Internet]. Geneva: World Health Organization; 2017. [cited June 15 2023]. Available at: https://www.ncbi.nlm.nih.gov/books/NBK493081/.
9. Roberts JM, Rich-Edwards JW, McElrath TF, Garmire L, Myatt L, for the Global Pregnancy Collaboration. Subtypes of preeclampsia: recognition and determining clinical usefulness. Hypertension. 2021;77(5):1430–41.
10. Vigil-De Gracia P, Vargas C, Sánchez J, Collantes-Cubas J. Preeclampsia: narrative review for clinical use. Heliyon. 2023;9(3):e14187.
11. Haram K, Svendsen E, Abildgaard U. The HELLP syndrome: clinical issues and management. A review. BMC Pregnancy Childbirth. 2009;9(1):8.
12. Bonet M, Brizuela V, Abalos E, Cuesta C, Baguiya A, Chamillard M, et al. Frequency and management of maternal infection in health facilities in 52 countries (GLOSS): a 1-week inception cohort study. Lancet Glob Health. 2020;8(5):e661–71.
13. Singer M, Deutschman CS, Seymour CW, Shankar-Hari M, Annane D, Bauer M, et al. The third international consensus definitions for sepsis and septic shock (Sepsis-3). JAMA. 2016;315(8):801.
14. Dolea C, Abouzahr C. Global burden of obstructed labour in the year 2000. Evidence and Information for Policy [Internet] 2000 Jan [cited 2023 June 16]; Available from: https://www.researchgate.net/publication/238084600_Global_burden_of_obstructed_labour_in_the_year_2000/citation/download
15. World Health Organization. Abortion: key facts [Internet]. World Health Organization; (Fact Sheets). Available from: https://www.who.int/news-room/fact-sheets/detail/abortion
16. Grimes DA, Benson J, Singh S, Romero M, Ganatra B, Okonofua FE, Shah IH. Unsafe abortion: the preventable pandemic. Lancet. 2006;368(9550):1908–19.

17. United Nations Children's Fund (UNICEF). Antenatal care [Internet]. United Nations Children's Fund (UNICEF); 2020 May. Available from: https://gdc.unicef.org/resource/antenatal-care#:~:text=Globally%2C%20while%2086%20per%20cent,at%20least%20four%20antenatal%20visits

18. World Health Organization. Antenatal care coverage – at least four visits (%) [Internet]. The Global Health Observatory; Available from: https://www.who.int/data/gho/indicator-metadata-registry/imr-details/80

19. Omer S, Zakar R, Zakar MZ, Fischer F. The influence of social and cultural practices on maternal mortality: a qualitative study from South Punjab, Pakistan. Reprod Health. 2021;18(1):97.

20. Black R, Laxminarayan R, Temmerman M, Walker N, editors. Disease control priorities, third edition (volume 2): reproductive, maternal, newborn, and child health [Internet]. The World Bank; 2016 [cited 2023 July 12]. Chapter 7. Available from: http://elibrary.worldbank.org/doi/book/10.1596/978-1-4648-0348-2

21. Pathmanathan I, Liljestrand J, editors. Investing in maternal health: learning from Malaysia and Sri Lanka, Health, nutrition, and population series. Washington, D.C: World Bank; 2003. 182 p.

22. Life For African Mothers. Making birth safer in sub-Saharan Africa [internet]. 2023. Available from: https://www.lifeforafricanmothers.org/

23. World Health Organization. Family planning/contraception methods: key facts [Internet]. World Health Organization; 2020 Nov. Available from: https://www.who.int/news-room/fact-sheets/detail/family-planning-contraception.

24. Lori JR, Perosky J, Munro-Kramer ML, Veliz P, Musonda G, Kaunda J, et al. Maternity waiting homes as part of a comprehensive approach to maternal and newborn care: a cross-sectional survey. BMC Pregnancy Childbirth. 2019 Dec;19(1):228.

Chapter 10
Importance of Gender Equality

Francesca L. Evans and Stephanie L. Rowlands

10.1   What Is Gender Equality?

Gender equality refers to access to rights or opportunities irrespective of gender. Gender is the socially constructed characteristics of men and women which includes gender roles, behavioural and social norms. Sex, on the other hand, refers to the physiological and biological characteristics of females, males and intersex people such as chromosomes, hormones and reproductive organs [1] (Fig. 10.1).

Despite universal healthcare being a human right, gender can influence the quality and accessibility of healthcare, and women often face multiple barriers to accessing healthcare services (Fig. 10.2). Furthermore, inequalities experienced by women and girls affect their social determinants of health.

Harmful gender norms can also negatively impact men as beliefs related to masculinity can prevent men from seeking help for mental and physical health issues. Rigid gender norms may have adverse effects on transgender individuals whose sex assigned at birth does not align with their perceived gender identity [1].

10.2   The Gender Inequality Index

The Gender Inequality Index is used to measure the level of gender inequality within a country. It takes three aspects of human development into account:.

Reproductive Health	Empowerment	Economic Status

F. L. Evans (✉) · S. L. Rowlands
School of Medicine, Cardiff University, Cardiff, UK
e-mail: rowlandssl1@cardiff.ac.uk

© The Author(s), under exclusive license to Springer Nature
Switzerland AG 2024
A. Fiander, G. Fry (eds.), *A Healthcare Students Introduction to Global Health*,
https://doi.org/10.1007/978-3-031-66563-9_10

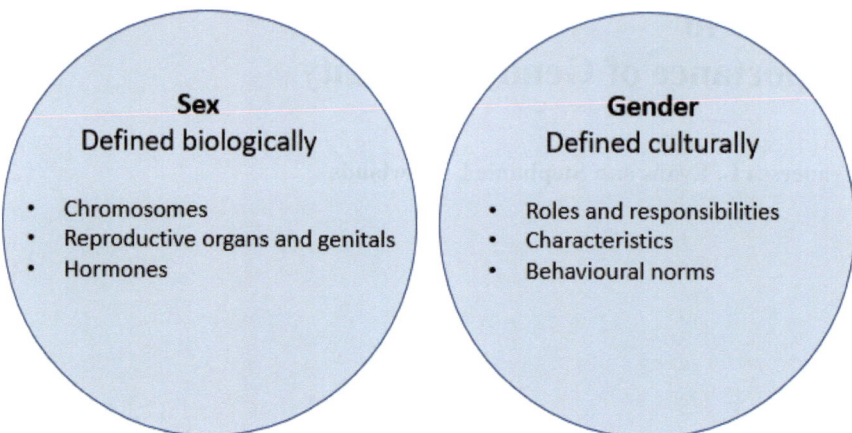

Fig. 10.1 Differences between sex and gender

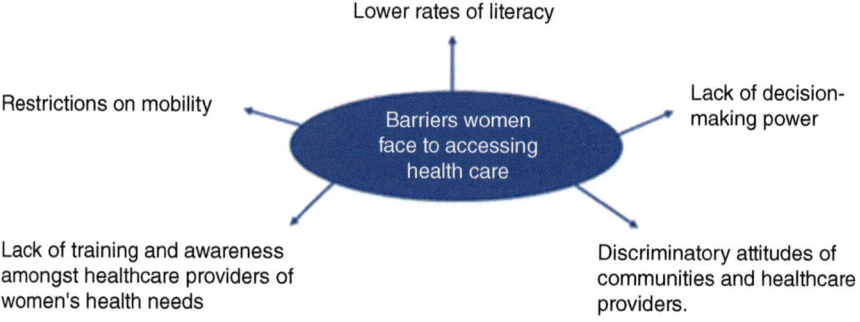

Fig. 10.2 Barriers women face to accessing healthcare

- Reproductive health is measured by maternal mortality ratio (MMR) and includes adolescent birth rates.
- Empowerment is measured by the proportion of parliamentary seats occupied by females and proportion of females and males over 25 in secondary education.
- Economic status is measured by labour force participation of men and women over 15 [3].

An equality score of 0–1 is generated based on the three aspects of human development above. A higher score therefore indicates greater gender inequality within that country. African and South Asian countries have the highest Gender Inequality Index scores globally (see Fig. 10.3).

Gender Inequality Index, 2021

This index covers three dimensions: reproductive health, empowerment, and economic status. Scores are between 0-1 and higher values indicate higher inequalities.

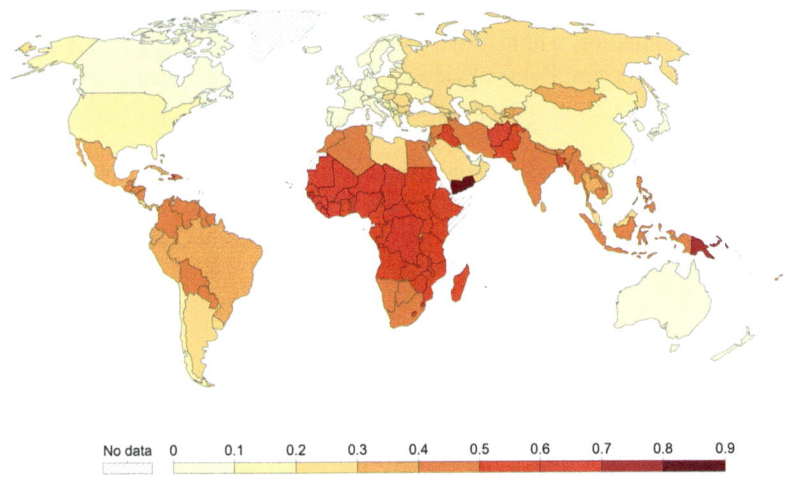

Source: UNDP, Human Development Report (2021-22)   OurWorldInData.org/economic-inequality-by-gender • CC BY

Fig. 10.3 Gender inequality index [2]. (Permission from: Figure available open access under the creative commons BY License (details at: https://ourworldindata.org/faqs#can-i-use-or-reproduce-your-data))

10.3 The 5 P's

The 5 P's outline the main reasons for poor health in women, especially in low resource countries (LRCs) [4]:

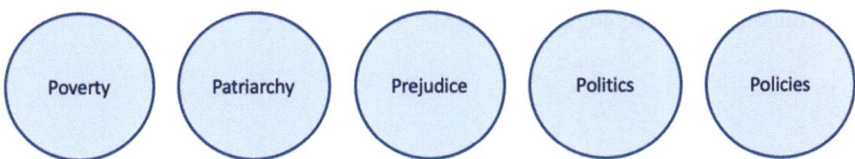

1. *Poverty*

   Women in LRCs do not often have access to their own finances. Therefore, they cannot pay to access healthcare, medicines or travel to hospital.
2. *Patriarchy*

   Men hold the vast majority of positions of power. Child marriage, gender-based violence and honour killings all cause women's health to suffer at the hands of men.
3. *Prejudice*

There is stigma surrounding living with HIV, having an abortion and being pregnant in adolescence. This stigma can prevent women seeking help for fear of judgement.

4. *Political views*

    Pro-life standpoints within governments prevent funds being put into safe and legal abortion services. Political views can also curb proper teaching on contraception, resulting in unwanted pregnancies.

5. *Policies*

    Abortion is illegal in some countries which forces women to seek out unsafe abortions. In addition, confidentiality laws in some countries allow an individual's HIV status to be disclosed without their consent. This can put women off seeing a healthcare professional.

10.4 Abuse of Women

10.4.1 Female Genital Mutilation

Female genital mutilation (FGM) is any procedure that involves partial or total removal of, or injury of, the external female genitalia. FGM is practised in many countries across the globe for several cultural reasons (Table 10.1). Over 200 million women and girls have undergone FGM, predominantly in countries in Africa, Asia and the middle East, and it is most often performed on young girls before the age of 15. Unfortunately, there are many complications of FGM including immediate complications from the procedure such as infection, haemorrhage and sepsis. Longer-term complications include keloid scars, abscesses, subfertility, recurrent urinary tract infections (UTIs) as well as sexual complications. Furthermore, FGM can complicate labour and the post-partum period and hinder vaginal examinations with regards to gynaecological health [5].

Table 10.1 The various reasons FGM is performed [6]

Psychosexual	Social and religious	Hygiene and aesthetic	Myths
Increased male sexual pleasure as often the vaginal orifice is made smaller	FGM is often considered a right of passage into womanhood and part of cultural heritage	The external female genitalia are considered dirty in some cultures and are removed to promote hygiene.	Fertility is thought to be improved
Prevention of female pleasure due to removal of the clitoris is thought to reduce female promiscuity and maintain chastity until marriage	Some communities believe that FGM is required according to their religion	Removal of the external female genitalia is considered more aesthetically pleasing	Child survival is thought to be improved.

10.4.2 Sexual Assault and Violence

The World Health Organisation (WHO) reports that globally about one in three women have been subjected to either physical and/or sexual violence in their lifetime. Most abuse occurs by an intimate partner, and across many countries, the law does not protect women against rape in marriage. Furthermore, child and forced marriages are still widely practised, particularly in conflict-affected areas. Globally, 20% of girls are married before reaching age 18, but in some countries, this is as high as 40%. By definition, a child marriage is a forced marriage as children cannot consent to marriage [7].

10.5 Women's Health

Women's health is an important aspect of gender equality and tends to be an under-appreciated area of healthcare.

10.5.1 Abortion Laws and Family Planning

The World Health Organisation (WHO) has recorded the number of abortions performed in all countries and found that the legality of abortion across the world has very little effect on abortion rates. Legal status does however impact women's access to safe abortions carried out by qualified health care professionals. In countries where abortion is illegal, the impact can be catastrophic; unsafe abortions account for up to 13% of maternal death usually as a result of sepsis, haemorrhage and surgical complications [8].

The laws relating to abortion are hugely diverse across the globe (Fig. 10.4). There are currently many countries where all abortions are illegal in all circumstances and many more that only allow abortion in extreme circumstances where the pregnancy threatens the mother's life.

With the status of abortions being illegal in many countries and limited in many others, one would hope that women have universal accesses to family planning advice and contraceptives to compensate. Unfortunately, this is not the case, and 270 billon women of reproductive age have an unmet need for contraception (Fig. 10.5). Use of contraception is beneficial with regards to health as infant mortality is evidenced to be increased when births are spaced less than 2 years apart. Furthermore, use of contraceptive empowers women to make reproductive choices and offers the potential to prioritise other opportunities such as work and education [10].

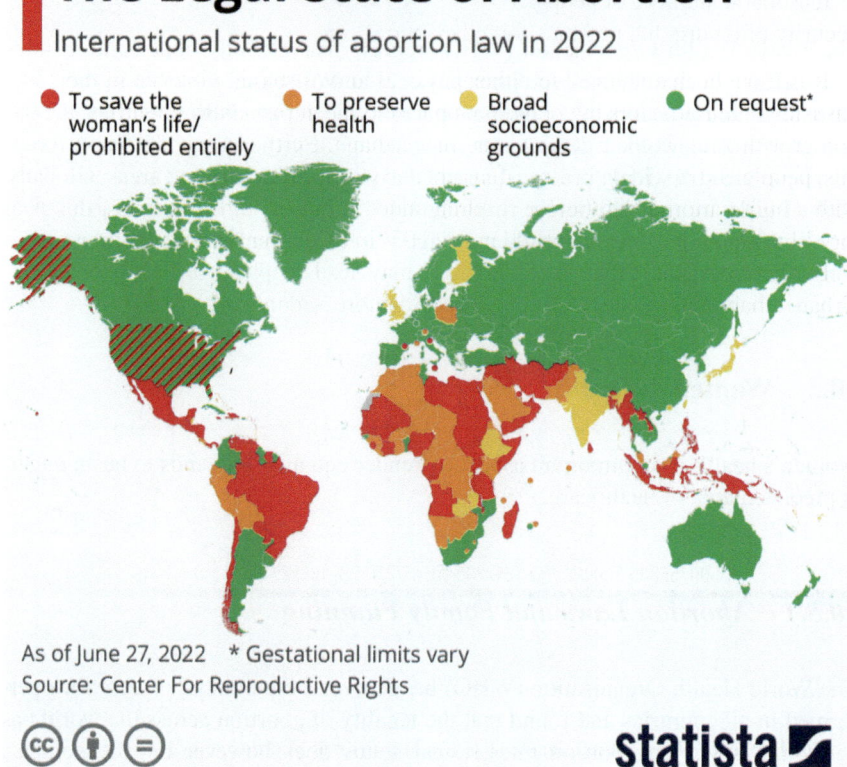

Fig. 10.4 International status of abortion law in 2022 [9]. (Permission from: Available under the Creative Commons License CC BY-ND 3.0 (details at: https://www.statista.com/chart/13680/the-legal-status-of-abortion-worldwide/))

10.5.2 Maternal and Neonatal Mortality

Women's pregnancy and childbirth outcomes vary greatly across the world (Fig. 10.6). In 2020, there were 800 daily preventable maternal deaths during pregnancy and childbirth. Ninety-four per cent of all maternal deaths occur in low- and lower-middle-income countries (LMICs) [12].

During the course of the pregnancy and childbirth, 15% of women develop complications needing emergency interventions, and it has been proposed that there are three types of delay that contribute to a high maternal mortality (Fig. 10.7). Many of these deaths are preventable; access to trained healthcare professionals before, during and after childbirth can save the lives of women and new-borns [13].

Share of women whose family planning needs are met, 2020
The proportion of women of reproductive age (15-49 years) who are currently using at least one modern
contraceptive¹ method, out of the total population of women who have demand for family planning² methods.

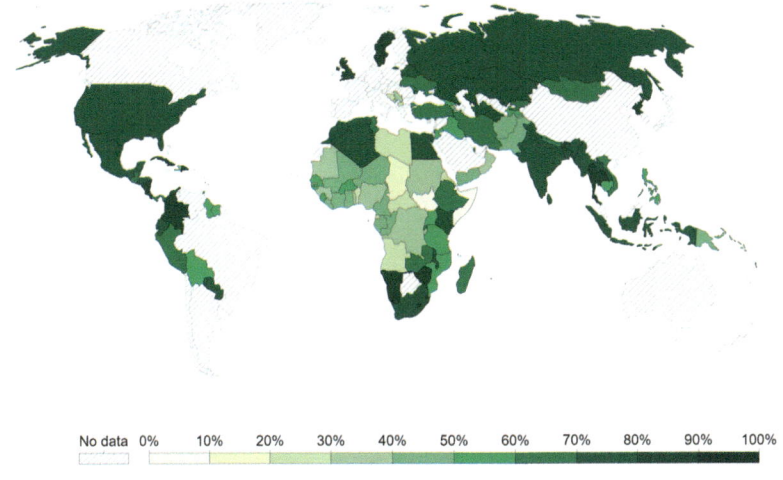

No data 0%   10%   20%   30%   40%   50%   60%   70%   80%   90%   100%

Source: Data from multiple sources compiled by the UN   OurWorldInData.org/fertility-rate • CC BY

1. **Modern contraception**: Modern contraceptive methods include: oral hormonal pills, intrauterine devices (IUDs), male or female condoms, emergency
contraception, implant, sterilization, injectables, and vaginal barrier methods.

2. **Family planning**: Family planning allows people to attain their desired number of children, if any, and to determine the spacing of their pregnancies. It
is achieved through use of contraceptive methods and the treatment of infertility.

Fig. 10.5 Demand for family planning satisfied by modern methods 2020 [11]. (Permission from:
Figure available open access under the creative commons BY License (details at: https://ourworld-
indata.org/faqs#can-i-use-or-reproduce-your-data))

10.6 Gender Bias in Health Research

Female scientists are underrepresented in research, making up 30% of the world's
researchers. This is particularly seen in higher-ranking positions within companies
and organisations. This has subsequent effects on the funding of research. Women's
research proposals are less likely to receive funding, especially if the focus of the
research is on a medical condition that only affects females. Funding into endome-
triosis is an example of this systemic gender bias. Despite the fact that endometrio-
sis affects 10% of women, making it as common as diabetes, it receives minimal
funding and only a fraction of that invested in diabetes research, likely because the
condition only affects females [15].

Gender bias is also seen in study design itself where research is largely conducted on groups of males, and the findings are then applied to females. The roles
of sex and gender are often disregarded within data analysis. Historically, it was
assumed that men and women are not fundamentally different other than in size and
reproductive organs. However, researchers have found differences between the
sexes in terms of organs, tissues and even at a cellular level. The majority of human

Maternal mortality ratio, 2020

The maternal mortality ratio is the number of women who die from pregnancy-related causes while pregnant or within 42 days of pregnancy termination per 100,000 live births.

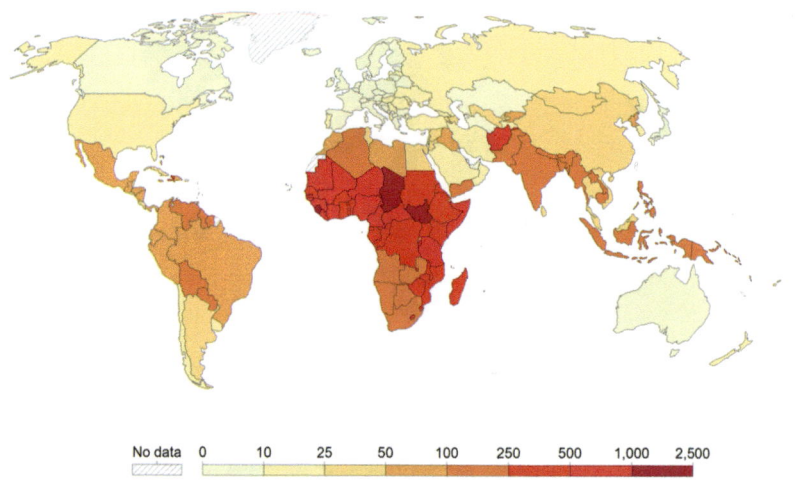

No data 0   10   25   50   100   250   500   1,000   2,500

Source: Gapminder (2010); WHO (2019); OECD (2022)   OurWorldInData.org/maternal-mortality • CC BY

Fig. 10.6 Maternal mortality ratio 2020 [14]. (Permission from: Figure available open access under the creative commons BY License (details at: https://ourworldindata.org/faqs#can-i-use-or-reproduce-your-data))

Fig. 10.7 The three delays that contribute to high maternal mortality in low resource countries

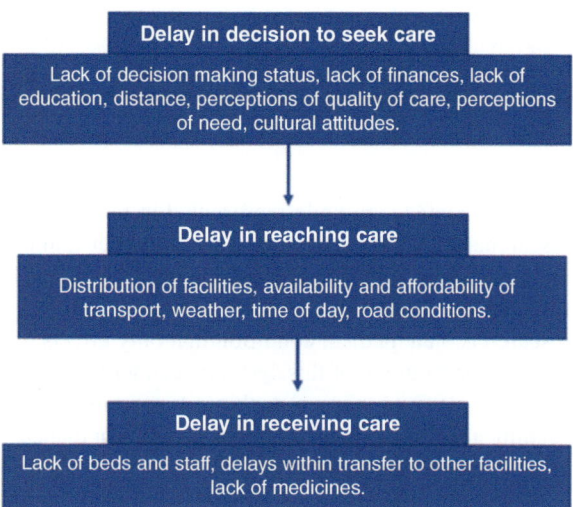

diseases also show sex differences in the course, severity and prevalence. It is therefore vital that we do not ignore the findings in 50% of the population as this inevitably leads to gender health inequality [16].

For example, in a 2016 Human immunodeficiency virus (HIV) study, women constituted just 19.2% of participants in antiretroviral studies and 38.1% in vaccination studies. This is in spite of the fact that 55% of HIV-positive adults are female. Given that we know women experience different clinical symptoms and complications of HIV, it is vital that they are appropriately and fairly represented within research [17].

10.7   The Wider Impact of Gender Inequality

Gender inequalities within healthcare do not only affect women themselves, but also have implications for their children, the climate and the economy.

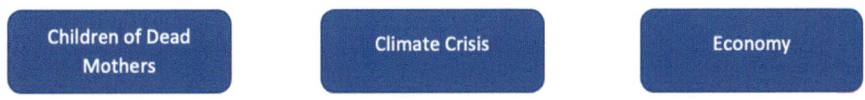

Impact of gender inequality on existing children of dead mothers:

- As mentioned in the previous paragraphs, maternal mortality rates are thought to be associated with gender inequality and delays to accessing correct healthcare.
- When women die due to pregnancy-related complications, they often leave behind older children.
- These children are more likely to drop out of school, and their daughters are more likely to have teenage pregnancies (Hub Cymru Africa 2020) [4].
- These children are also 15 times more likely to die than children whose mothers are still alive [18].

Impact of gender inequality on the climate crisis:

- Gender inequality results in fewer women being educated.
- Women are more likely to have large families if they are not in education or have had reduced access to education.
- Having more children increases the size of the population which increases greenhouse gas emissions [19].

Impact of gender inequality on the economy:

- Uneducated women are unlikely to seek high-paying jobs and are more likely to remain unemployed.
- Educating women would empower them to seek better employment which would contribute to economic growth [19].

10.7.1   The Need for Women in Power

There is a male dominance in government leadership (Fig. 10.8). Given that men possess the majority of power, it is vital to have men as allies in promoting systemic changes towards gender equality. However, it is equally as important to increase female participation in politics as studies have shown that women leaders are more likely to prioritise 'women's issues' as well as education and healthcare compared to men [20].

10.8   Targets for the Future—Sustainable Development Goals (SDGs)

From what has been mentioned in this chapter, it is clear that gender equality needs to be achieved in order to improve the lives of many, but how will we do this? The sustainable development goals were outlined by the United Nations (UN) in 2015 and are a set of 17 goals to achieve a more sustainable future for all by 2030 (Fig. 10.9).

Some of the SDGs look to achieve gender equality [23]:

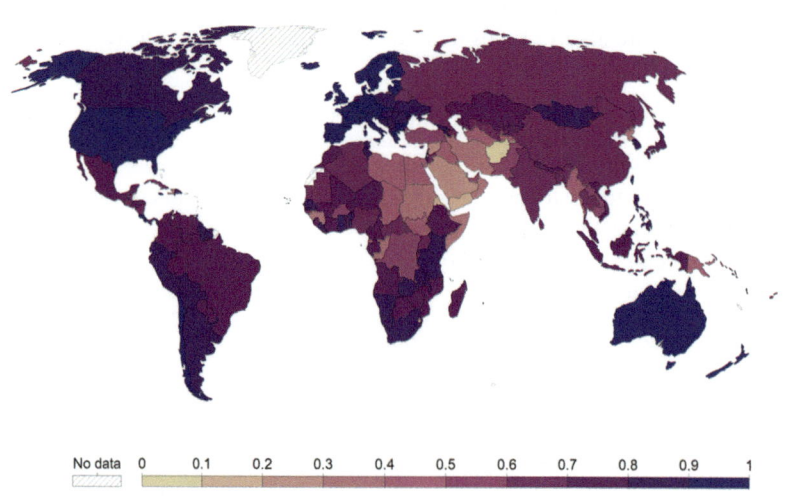

Women's political empowerment, 2022

Based on the expert assessments and index by V-Dem. It captures the extent to which women enjoy civil liberties, can participate in civil society, and are represented in politics. It ranges from 0 to 1 (most empowered).

No data   0   0.1   0.2   0.3   0.4   0.5   0.6   0.7   0.8   0.9   1

Source: OWID based on V-Dem (v13)   OurWorldInData.org/women-rights • CC BY

Fig. 10.8 Women's political empowerment [21]. (Permission from: Figure available open access under the creative commons BY License (details at: https://ourworldindata.org/faqs#can-i-use-or-reproduce-your-data))

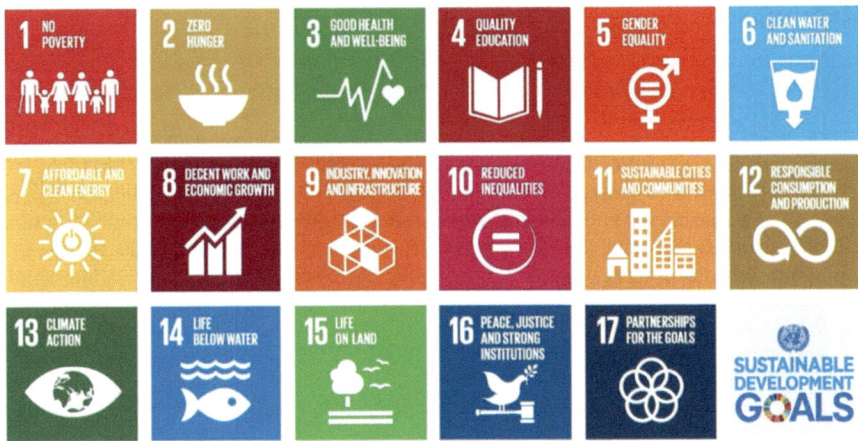

Fig. 10.9 Sustainable development goals [22]. (Permission from: Figure available open access under the creative commons BY License (details at: https://sdg-tracker.org/))

SDG 4—Quality Education for All

Targets
- Ensure all girls and boys have equal access to primary and secondary education
- Ensure all girls and boys have access to quality early childhood development
- Ensure equal access for all women and men to quality tertiary education
- Eliminate gender disparities in education

SDG 5—To Achieve Gender Equality and Empower All Women and Girls

Targets
- Eliminate discrimination, violence and harmful practices against women and girls everywhere
- Provide women with equal opportunities for leadership in political, economic and public life
- To ensure universal access to sexual and reproductive health services
- To undertake reforms to give women and men equal rights to economic resource

10.9   How Can We Achieve these Goals?

Since men currently make up the vast majority of those in positions of power, it is important that men work as allies with women to work towards gender equality. The content of this chapter has outlined why gender equality should be in everyone's best interests. It is important to educate national leaders on these points, so that legislation can be changed to help males and females become more equal, empower women and protect women's health as a result.

References

1. WHO. Gender and health. https://www.who.int/health-topics/gender#tab=tab_1 (2023). Accessed 3 June 2023.
2. OurWorldinData. Gender inequality index 2021. https://ourworldindata.org/grapher/gender-inequality-index-from-the-human-development-report (2021). Accessed 3 June 2023.
3. UnitedNationsDevelopmentProgramme. Gender inequality index (GII). http://hdr.undp.org/en/content/gender-inequality-index-gii (2020). Accessed 21 Apr 2021.
4. HubCymruAfrica. Sexual reproductive health and equality – #HealthForAll2020. 2020.
5. Rymer J. Female genital mutilation. Curr Obstet Gynaecol. 2003;13(3):185–90. https://doi.org/10.1016/S0957-5847(03)00004-0.
6. Braddy CM, Files JA. Female genital mutilation: cultural awareness and clinical considerations. J Midwifery Womens Health. 2007;52(2):158–63. https://doi.org/10.1016/j.jmwh.2006.11.001.
7. WHO. Violence against women. https://www.who.int/news-room/fact-sheets/detail/violence-against-women (2021). Accessed 27 June 2023.
8. WHO. Abortion. https://www.who.int/news-room/fact-sheets/detail/abortion (2021). Accessed 27 June 2023.
9. Armstrong M. The legal status of abortion worldwide. https://www.statista.com/chart/13680/the-legal-status-of-abortion-worldwide/ (2022). Accessed 03 June 2023.
10. WHO. Family planning/contraception methods. https://www.who.int/news-room/fact-sheets/detail/family-planning-contraception (2020). Accessed 27 June 2023.
11. OurWorldinData. Share of women whose family planning needs are met, 2020. https://ourworldindata.org/grapher/share-of-married-women-ages-15-49-years-whose-need-for-family-planning-is-satisfied (2020). Accessed 3 June 2023.
12. WHO. Trends in materna mortality 2000–2020: estimates by WHO, UNICEF, UNFPA, World Bank Group and UNESDA/Population Division. https://www.who.int/publications/i/item/9789240068759 (2023). Accessed 27 June 2023.
13. Mgawadere F, Unkels R, Kazembe A, van den Broek N. Factors associated with maternal mortality in Malawi: application of the three delays model. BMC Pregnancy Childbirth. 2017;17(1):219. https://doi.org/10.1186/s12884-017-1406-5.
14. OurWorldinData. Maternal mortality ratio, 2020. https://ourworldindata.org/grapher/maternal-mortality (2020). Accessed 3 June 2023.
15. Cislak A, Formanowicz M, Saguy T. Bias against research on gender bias. Scientometrics. 2018;115:189–200. https://doi.org/10.1007/s11192-018-2667-0.
16. Holdcroft A. Gender bias in research: how does it affect evidence based medicine? London: SAGE Publications Sage UK; 2007. p. 2–3.
17. Curno MJ, Rossi S, Hodges-Mameletzis I, Johnston R, Price MA, Heidari S. A systematic review of the inclusion (or exclusion) of women in HIV research: from clinical studies of antiretrovirals and vaccines to cure strategies. J Acquir Immune Defic Syndr. 2016;71(2):181–8. https://doi.org/10.1097/qai.0000000000000842.
18. Houle B, Clark SJ, Kahn K, Tollman S, Yamin AE. The impacts of maternal mortality and cause of death on children's risk of dying in rural South Africa: evidence from a population based surveillance study (1992-2013). Reprod Health. 2015;12(1):S7. https://doi.org/10.1186/1742-4755-12-S1-S7.
19. ProjectDrawdown. Health and education. https://ourworldindata.org/grapher/women-political-empowerment (2021). Accessed 21 Apr 2021.
20. Cowper-Coles M. Women political leaders: the impact of gender on democracy. https://www.kcl.ac.uk/giwl/research/women-political-leaders-the-impact-of-gender-on-democracy (2023). Accessed 3 July 2023.
21. OurWorldinData. Women's political empowerment, 2022. https://ourworldindata.org/grapher/women-political-empowerment (2022). Accessed 3 June 2023.

22. Ritchie R, Mispy O-O. Measuring progress towards the Sustainable Development Goals. https://sdg-tracker.org/ (2018). Accessed 3 June 2023.
23. UnitedNations. The 17 goals. https://sdgs.un.org/goals (2021). Accessed 21 Apr 2021.

Chapter 11
Child Health in Low-Resource Countries

Florence Vincent and Damien Carroll

11.1 Background

11.1.1 Definition of Low-Resource Countries (LRCs)

The World Bank defines LRCs as countries with weaker economies. Due to poor economic health, LRCs often have worse health outcomes for their populations compared to countries with a higher gross national income per capita.

11.1.2 Importance of Child Health

The first month of a child's life is their most vulnerable stage. The World Health Organisation (WHO) estimates that in 2019 there were 2.4 million neonatal or perinatal (<28 days old) deaths worldwide. This makes up almost half of the estimated 5.2 million deaths in children under five years of age. Infant deaths (aged one month to one year) accounted for 1.5 million deaths in 2019 [2].

F. Vincent (✉) · D. Carroll
Royal Free London NHS Trust, London, UK

11.1.3 Causes of Death and Underlying Factors Contributing to Child Mortality

Of the 2.4 million neonatal deaths in 2019, around one million new-borns died within the first 24 hours of their life. Preterm birth, intrapartum-related complications such as asphyxia, infections and congenital birth defects are the leading causes of neonatal deaths. Studies have shown that many of these deaths are preventable [3]. In England and Wales in 2021, the neonatal mortality rate was 2.7 deaths per 1000 live births. South Sudan had the highest neonatal mortality rate in 2021 at 39.6 deaths per 1000 live births. Even after they have overcome the risks of the first month, infants (one month to one year) and children (one to five years) in LRCs are then exposed to several other life-threatening diseases. Child mortality decreases after the first month falling from an average 18 deaths per 1000 live births (neonatal), to 11 (infant) and to 10 (children) [4]. Pneumonia, diarrhoea and malaria are the three leading causes of death in children under five in LRCs. This chapter focuses on these causes and the poverty-linked corresponding social, environmental and cultural factors that pose the greatest burden of disease in child mortality.

11.2 Pneumonia

11.2.1 Overview

Pneumonia is the leading infectious cause of deaths in children worldwide. The WHO reports that pneumonia killed 740,180 children under five in 2019. This accounted for 14% of all child deaths worldwide. Bacterial and viral pneumonia are largely preventable with vaccination. Once recognised, it is a treatable condition. In LRCs, children lack access to appropriate antibiotics and oxygen and have lower rates of completing their childhood vaccination schedule. The prevalence of pneumonia-related mortality is heightened in LRCs due to children's weakened immune systems from, for example, inadequate nutrition or infants who have not been exclusively breastfed [5, 6].

11.2.2 Causes

Pneumonia is caused by bacterial, viral or fungal pathogens. *Haemophilus influenzae* type B (Hib), *Streptococcus pneumoniae* (Pneumococcus) and the *Influenzae* virus are pathogens that are responsible for over a third of severe episodes of pneumonia and two-thirds of childhood mortalities relating to acute respiratory infections [7]. These are all pathogens that are preventable through vaccination. A study published in the Lancet in 2018 looked at how the disease burden of pneumococcus and Hib affected child mortality and how it has changed since the widespread use of vaccines for these infections [8]. They estimate that between 2000 and 2015, pneumococcal and Hib deaths in children decreased by 51% and 90%, respectively. Most of these deaths come from a small number of large countries in Asia and Africa where the vaccines were only introduced towards the end of the study period, some with limited uptake. Suboptimal housing conditions are due to air pollution from indoor fumes and gases used for cooking. Furthermore, overcrowding increases transmission of respiratory pathogens via airborne routes.

11.2.3 Treatment and Prevention

The WHO and the United Nations International Children's Emergency Fund (UNICEF) are working in collaboration to publish an Integrated Global Action Plan for the Prevention and Control of Pneumonia and Diarrhoea to reduce deaths from pneumonia [9]. Their aims are three-fold:

- *Protection*—Breastfeeding and vitamin A supplementation are effective measures that protect children from getting pneumonia.
- *Prevention*—By vaccinating children, they are less likely to acquire the disease. This is effective alongside the minimisation of risk factors (e.g., Human Immunodeficiency Virus (HIV) infection, malnutrition, poor sanitation, and air pollution) so that the child has an optimally functioning immune system.
- *Treatment*—If a child does get pneumonia, they have the right to essential care including appropriate antibiotics and oxygen.

Families of higher economic status are more likely to complete their children's vaccination doses as well as receive antibiotics for pneumonia than poorer families. This inequality across society is more pronounced in LRCs compared to upper and middle-income countries [10].

11.3 Preterm Birth Complications

11.3.1 Overview

A child that is born alive before 37 weeks' gestation is defined as preterm. Preterm birth complications (e.g., birth defects, underdeveloped organs, and immune system) are the leading cause of deaths in the neonatal period [11]. Preterm birth complications contribute significantly towards child morbidity and mortality in LRCs. The WHO estimates that in 2020 there were 13.4 million preterm babies, representing over 10% of births [12]. Almost one million children were estimated to have died in 2019 due to complications related to being preterm. Disparities in mortality rates exist between countries, with nine out of ten babies born before 28 weeks surviving in high-income countries compared to one in ten in LRCs [13]. The outcomes are improved in high-income countries due to access to skilled birth attendants, improved neonatal and prenatal care and neonatal intensive care units (NICU).

11.3.2   Causes, Risk Factors, and Consequences

Preterm birth can be spontaneous or provider-initiated, for example when medical factors such as infection or obstetric complications necessitate the early induction of labour or a caesarean section. Preterm birth complications in LRCs are caused by a range of risk factors and have severe consequences for both the infants and their families. Limited access to healthcare, inadequate prenatal care, maternal malnutrition and vulnerability to and lack of treatment of infections are examples of how resource constraints in LRCs contribute to the low preterm survival rate. Moreover, preterm birth poses a risk of long-term disability due to compromised neurodevelopment and respiratory complications. This results in a high burden of disease as the family suffers chronic socioeconomic inequalities secondary to their child's disability [14].

11.3.3   Reducing Preterm Mortality

The approach taken by the WHO to reducing preterm mortality is two-fold: preventing preterm birth and improving new-born care. This involves reducing maternal risk factors and ensuring early detection and treatment of infections, thus preventing the need for provider-initiated preterm birth unless medically necessary. Simultaneously, the WHO advocates for improving new-born care by promoting breastfeeding, kangaroo mother care and well-equipped NICUs (e.g., access to oxygen via continuous positive airway pressure masks for preterm babies in acute respiratory distress). By addressing these areas, the WHO seeks to minimise the disparities in survival of preterm babies between LRCs and their higher-income counterparts.

11.4   Diarrhoeal Disease

11.4.1   Overview

Diarrhoea is defined as the passing of three or more loose stools per day or more than usual for the individual person. Diarrhoea is the second most common cause of death in young children less than five years of age [15]. Diarrhoea can be caused by a variety of pathogens that are often spread via the faecal-oral route. In LRCs, children under three years old experience on average three episodes of diarrhoea every year [15].

Diarrhoea can cause an excess loss of electrolytes and fluids from the body which the affected person can often struggle to replace. This leads to dehydration. Diarrhoea also can exacerbate malnutrition, which in turn can make an individual more susceptible to further episodes of diarrhoea.

11.4.2   Causes

The two most common pathogens are *Rotavirus* and *Escherichia coli* [16]. Other causes include *Cholera, Campylobacter* and *Salmonella*.

Most strains of *E. coli* are harmless and are contained in the lower intestine as part of the normal gut flora. However, the Shiga toxin-producing *E. coli* (STEC) is a bacterium that has the potential to cause significant diarrhoea. The most significant serotype is *E. coli* O157:H7 in health surveillance/outbreaks. For most of the cases, it is a self-limiting infection. However, it can have life-threatening complications such as haemolytic uremic syndrome. The sources of outbreaks of STEC are usually due to raw or undercooked meat or raw milk. STEC can be eliminated from food products by thoroughly heating food. The WHO has created some guidance called 'five ways to safer food' to provide information to prevent transmission [17].

Internationally, rotavirus infection was the leading cause of diarrhoeal deaths, accounting for nearly a fifth of deaths from diarrhoea in 2019 [16]. Rotavirus caused a higher death burden in LRCs in Africa and Asia [16]. There is a large amount of diversity among different strains of the virus, but most rotaviruses causing diarrhoeal illness are thought to belong to serogroup A (but B and C may also cause disease in humans) [18]. It is easily spread as in an infected individual the rotavirus sheds in high concentrations in faeces and vomit. Rotaviruses are mainly transmitted from person-to-person through the faecal-oral route, but transmission may also occur indirectly through contaminated objects. The infective period is one to three weeks. Asymptomatic carriers are common.

11.4.3   Treatment and Prevention

The most important management regarding all causes of diarrhoea is rehydration and replacement of electrolytes. This can be achieved in mild cases with oral rehydration solution. In severe or resistant cases, fluid may have to be provided intravenously. Improving dietary intake to ensure that it provides adequate nutrition also plays a role. Zinc supplements have been shown to reduce the duration of a diarrhoeal episode and show a reduction in stool volume [19].

To reduce complications of diarrhoea, the provision of trained health professionals to review and effectively manage severe episodes is important.

Education plays a key role with an emphasis on the importance of personal hygiene and handwashing. It also involves providing resources, so that people are aware of how these infections are spread as well as educating them on measures to reduce transmission. Breastfeeding infants has been shown to reduce the chance of getting diarrhoeal illnesses and the severity of diarrhoea symptoms. The WHO currently recommends (when possible) to breastfeed infants for the first six months of their life [15].

There is also a role for vaccination. As of July 2020, more than 100 countries worldwide had introduced rotavirus vaccines in their national immunisation programmes [20].

The WHO has worked with charitable organisations and local governments to promote policies and direct investment into improving sanitation and access to clean water. There are also ongoing initiatives for research to develop new strategies to control breakouts of disease. The *Integrated Global Action Plan for the Prevention and Control of Pneumonia and Diarrhoea (GAPPD)*, by WHO/UNICEF, is one example aiming to make more efficient use of limited healthcare services for more effective outcomes [9].

11.5   Malaria

11.5.1   Overview

Malaria remains one of the biggest causes of death in children under five in LRCs. Of the 247 million cases estimated in 2021 worldwide, approximately 95% of these cases and 96% of deaths occurred in Africa [21]. Children under five accounted for around 80% of all malaria-related deaths in Africa. It is caused by the various types of *Plasmodium* parasites which use infected mosquitoes as their vector to infect humans. Children under five and those with compromised immune systems are at a higher risk of succumbing to a more severe infection and consequent death. Malaria is avoidable if you do not get bitten. Recognising positive cases and getting treatment early reduces mortality.

11.5.2 Causes

Among the five species of *Plasmodium* parasites that infect humans, two, namely *P. falciparum* and *P. vivax*, present the highest risk. Whilst *P. vivax* leads to more severe illness and mortality, *P. falciparum* poses the greatest danger as it is the most prevalent in Africa and is responsible for most malaria-related deaths. Once the human is infected with the parasite, it multiplies and destroys the human's red blood cells [22]. Initial symptoms are non-specific and include fever, headache and tiredness. These symptoms can progress to more severe symptoms and death.

11.5.3 Prevention and Treatment

Avoiding being bitten by the mosquito by using insecticide-treated nets (ITNs), indoor residual spraying (IRS) and mosquito larvae eradication are all forms of vector control. The 2022 world malaria report highlighted that due to the Covid-19 pandemic many efforts to control malaria were disrupted, with many countries running ITN distribution campaigns falling short on their targets [23]. Chemoprevention is recommended alongside vector control for at-risk populations (pregnant women, recently discharged patients and young children) in areas of moderate to high perennial malaria transmission. Prompt recognition and an accurate, parasitological diagnosis save lives and can minimise the spread of drug resistance. Artemisinin-based combination therapies are the most effective medication against *P. falciparum*. The world's first successful malaria vaccine is being rolled out to 12 low- and middle-income countries to deliver 18 million vaccines in 2023 to 2025 [24]. A combination of the aforementioned efforts alongside effective surveillance and response systems have allowed some countries to eliminate the disease [25].

11.6 Malnutrition

11.6.1 Causes and Consequences of Malnutrition

The term malnutrition refers to issues relating to imbalances in an individual's consumption of energy and/or nutrients. This imbalance may be under- or overconsumption of different food groups and micronutrients. Malnutrition can be divided into three conditions: undernutrition (stunting and wasting), micronutrient-related malnutrition (hidden hunger) and being overweight [26]. Being malnourished as a child results in poor growth, immunosuppression and impaired cognitive function. This puts the child at risk of serious health and socioeconomic consequences [27]. Concurrently, obesity is also becoming an issue in LRCs as families in poverty are unable to provide balanced diets with adequate food diversity and nutrition [28].

This leads to non-communicable diseases such as vasculopathic and metabolic diseases as well as some cancers in the future. Although there have been advancements over the last 20 years, it is estimated that globally a third of children under five fall into the 'undernutrition' or 'overweight' category. At least half of children under five are suffering from 'hidden hunger' as they are deficient in vitamins and other essential nutrients [28].

11.6.2 Maternal Nutrition

Starting at conception and continuing to adult life, maternal nutrition plays an important role in ensuring the child has the best possible start to their development. A malnourished mother's baby may be born prematurely, be at risk of perinatal complications and can contribute to foetal growth restriction [29]. Being deficient in essential nutrients or being anaemic during the pregnancy increases the risk of neonatal mortality. The 2019 report on 'The State of the World's Children' by UNICEF focussed on nutrition. It highlighted that less than 40% of children under six months of age are exclusively breastfed as is recommended by the WHO. After a child is weaned from breast milk, 'only one in five children aged six to 23 months from the poorest households and rural areas is fed the minimum recommended diverse diet for healthy growth and brain development'. [28]

With only limited improvements, the issue of maternal and child undernutrition continues to persist as a critical issue in global health.

11.7 Sanitation

11.7.1 Impact of Poor Sanitation in Child Health

Over the past 20 years, the world population that has access to safely managed sanitation services has increased from 33% to 57% [30]. However as of 2022, 3.5 billion people still lacked safely managed sanitation [30]. Poor sanitation increases the morbidity and mortality associated with faecal-oral infections. This has a significant impact on children in lower-income countries, who are at greatest risk of catching these infections and their associated symptoms and complications [31]. This has subsequently been shown to increase the severity and impact of malnutrition [31].

For young children living in these deprived communities, it disincentives further education as collecting water is prioritised over spending time at school. This burden of collecting water is disproportionately undertaken by young women and girls and can be hazardous in nature decreasing their safety and well-being [32].

There is also an environmental impact that results in a reduction in the potential recovery of water and nutrients from faecal waste; and the potential to mitigate water scarcity through safe use of wastewater [31].

A WHO study in 2012 calculated that for every US$1 invested in sanitation, this would result in a return of US$5.50 [33]. This was because of reduced healthcare costs, increased economic productivity and a reduction in premature deaths.

11.7.2   Waterborne Diseases and Infections

The WHO estimates that 4 per cent of all deaths worldwide are the result of waterborne diseases like diarrhoea, cholera, dysentery, typhoid and polio that all thrive in conditions without adequate sanitation systems [34]. All three infections discussed below (cholera, dysentery and typhoid) are spread via the faecal-oral route by the ingestion of contaminated food and drink.

Cholera is an acute diarrhoeal infection caused by the bacterium, *Vibrio cholerae*. It can affect people of all ages. In severe cases, it can be rapidly fatal. However, most cases can be successfully treated with oral rehydration solution. Severe cases will need urgent treatment with intravenous antibiotics and fluids. Annually, there can be up to four million cases of cholera, resulting in 143,000 deaths across the world [35].

Dysentery is caused by *Shigella* species. This involves the bacterium invading the colonic epithelium causing intense inflammation in the colon. This presents as bloody diarrhoea. The mainstay of treatment is rehydration. Antibiotics are reserved for severe cases due to concerns regarding resistance. One hundred eighty-eight million cases of shigellosis occur annually worldwide, with one million associated deaths [36].

Typhoid is caused by the bacterium *Salmonella typhi*. Typhoid fever can be treated with antibiotics. There is also the typhoid conjugate vaccine available. It is estimated that there are nine million cases of typhoid fever annually, and this results in about 110,000 deaths per year [37].

11.7.3   Promoting Access to Safe Water (WaSH)

Safe WaSH (water, sanitation and hygiene) is not only a prerequisite to health but has a greater impact as it contributes to dignity, school attendance and employment. Deaths attributed to diarrhoea due to poor WaSH were halved during the Millennium Development Goal (MDG) period (1990–2015). The considerable progress on water and sanitation provision is playing a key role in this [38].

Charitable organisations have worked closely with local communities to increase education regarding the importance of sanitation and clean water. This has focused on areas such as reducing open defecation and improving handwashing.

For future planning, it has been advised to invest strategically in building further safe drinking water systems. This is not as simple as allocating more funding. This also involves strengthening the existing systems in their capacity to plan and regulate water provision.

The progress observed in the past has shown a positive overall trend. However, this has been fragile and inequitable—the progress varies across the world and different environments (i.e., rural and urban areas). Factors such as climate change are making periods of rainfall unpredictable. This can exacerbate water insecurity and can limit water available to communities. Meanwhile, rapid urbanisation can put additional pressure on existing water infrastructure in cities. It is an added challenge to deliver water to the substantial number of people living in slums and informal communities.

11.8   Cultural Factors

11.8.1   Beliefs, Practices and Barriers to Health

Prompt recognition of a deterioration in a child's health and accessing appropriate healthcare services improves child health outcomes. Challenges such as cultural barriers to accessing healthcare are multiple, nuanced and vary between countries [39]. Barriers to health include communication breakdowns; misconceptions regarding orthodox medicine over traditional/herbal medicine; and living in rural areas with many dependent family members unable to be left alone [40]. Often, the hospital is perceived as the place patients only go to die. This perception forms a vicious cycle as there is a reluctance for family members to take their child to hospital. This results in late presentations, resulting in adverse health outcomes. Family hierarchy and gender inequality, for example the female members not being the financial decision-maker in taking a child or themselves to hospital, can also lead to delays in seeking healthcare [41]. It is imperative to comprehend and tackle these barriers in a culturally sensitive manner so that child and maternal health in LRCs can be improved in an impactful and sustainable way.

11.9   Future Directions for Improving Child Health in LRCs

11.9.1   Overview of SDGs

The Sustainable Developments Goals (SDGs) are a set of 17 goals established following the United Nations (UN) conference on Sustainable Development in Rio de Janeiro in 2012. The goals form a comprehensive and interlinking framework that all UN member states are to work towards by 2030 to end poverty as well as address environmental, political and economic issues [42]. Many of the goals and indicators are directly related to child health. SDG 2 aims for 'zero hunger' with stunting (defined as 'height-for-age' to be less than two standard deviations of the median of WHO Child Growth Standards) and prevalence of malnutrition among children under five being the main indicators. SDG 3 aims for 'good health and wellbeing'. This goal has 21 indicators; the most relevant to child health are child and maternal mortality rates, communicable disease incidence rates, proportion of population with access to health services and mortality rate attributed to household and ambient air pollution. SDG 6 aims for 'clean water and sanitation' with the proportion of the population with safe drinking water, sanitation and basic hand hygiene facilities being the indicators relevant to child health.

11.9.2 Progress Towards the Goals

The Sustainable Development Report in 2019 published that 'four years after the adoption of the SDGs and the Paris Agreement no country is on track to meeting all the goals'. [43] Since then, the world has changed. The 2022 report on SDGs highlights that the SDGs are in jeopardy due to a three-fold interlinked problem: conflict, Covid-19 and climate change [44]. Currently, the global community faces more conflict that the world has faced since the UN was created. Conflict, in particular the Ukraine crisis, has disrupted supply chains and caused economic instability. Recent setbacks also include the disruption of essential services due to the Covid-19 pandemic. As global temperatures rise due to the climate crisis, there are more medium- to large-scale natural disasters occurring worldwide, increasing the number of communities that are displaced. This has caused countries to perform particularly badly in SDG 2 and 3. Whilst the global coverage of drinking water, sanitation and hygiene services (SDG 6) has increased since 2015, it is not projected to meet the targets by 2030. The 2022 report states that to meet the SDG 6 by 2030, a four-fold increase in pace of progress is required. So, whilst there has been some progress in improving child health since the SDGs were established, more work needs to be done.

References

1. Convention on the rights of the child (1989) Treaty no. 27531. United Nations Treaty Series, vol 1577. Available at: https://treaties.un.org/doc/Publication/UNTS/Volume%201577/v1577.pdf
2. World Health Organization. Children: reducing mortality [Internet]. Who.int. World Health Organization: WHO; 2018. Available from: https://www.who.int/news-room/fact-sheets/detail/children-reducing-mortality.
3. Kruk ME, Gage AD, Joseph NT, Danaei G, García-Saisó S, Salomon JA. Mortality due to low-quality health systems in the universal health coverage era: a systematic analysis of amenable

deaths in 137 countries. Lancet. 2018;392(10160):2203–12. Available from: https://www.thelancet.com/journals/lancet/article/PIIS0140-6736(18)31668-4/fulltext

4. UNICEF. Neonatal mortality – UNICEF DATA [Internet]. UNICEF DATA 2023. Available from: https://data.unicef.org/topic/child-survival/neonatal-mortality/

5. UNICEF. Pneumonia in Children – UNICEF Data [Internet]. UNICEF DATA. 2022. Available from: https://data.unicef.org/topic/child-health/pneumonia/

6. World Health Organization. Pneumonia [Internet]. Who.int. World Health Organization: WHO; 2022. Available from: https://www.who.int/news-room/fact-sheets/detail/pneumonia.

7. Walker CLF, Rudan I, Liu L, Nair H, Theodoratou E, Bhutta ZA, et al. Global burden of childhood pneumonia and diarrhoea. The Lancet [Internet]. 2013;381(9875):1405–16. Available from: https://www.thelancet.com/journals/lancet/article/PIIS0140-6736(13)60222-6/fulltext?_eventId=login

8. Wahl B, O'Brien KL, Greenbaum A, Majumder A, Liu L, Chu Y, et al. Burden of Streptococcus pneumoniae and Haemophilus influenzae type b disease in children in the era of conjugate vaccines: global, regional, and national estimates for 2000–15. Lancet Glob Health. 2018;6(7):e744–57.

9. World Health Organisation, The United Nations Children's Fund. Ending Preventable Child Deaths from Pneumonia and Diarrhoea by 2025 – the integrated Global Action Plan for Pneumonia and Diarrhoea (GAPPD) Executive summary [Internet] 2013. Available from: https://apps.who.int/iris/bitstream/handle/10665/79207/WHO_FWC_MCA_13_01_eng.pdf

10. Kruk ME, Gage AD, Arsenault C, Jordan K, Leslie HH, Roder-DeWan S, et al. High-quality health systems in the Sustainable Development Goals era: time for a revolution. Lancet Global Health. 2018;6(11):e1196–252. Available from: https://www.thelancet.com/journals/langlo/article/PIIS2214-109X(18)30386-3/fulltext?_hsenc=p2ANqtz-9j71i5H1n10wxx2NBq1u-t2hYmpqLOEIQX0LxCN_gMwn8mnEO34buRcJMq9R0YratlH91E

11. Chawanpaiboon S, Vogel JP, Moller AB, Lumbiganon P, Petzold M, Hogan D, et al. Global, regional, and national estimates of levels of preterm birth in 2014: a systematic review and modelling analysis. Lancet Global Health. 2019;7(1):e37–46. Available from: https://www.thelancet.com/journals/langlo/article/PIIS2214-109X(18)30451-0/fulltext

12. World Health Organization. Preterm birth [Internet]. Preterm Birth. World Health Organization: WHO; 2023. Available from: https://www.who.int/news-room/fact-sheets/detail/preterm-birth

13. World Health Organization, Partnership for Maternal N and CH, Fund (UNICEF) UNC, Fund UNP. Born too soon: decade of action on preterm birth [Internet]. apps.who.int. World Health Organization; 2023. Available from: https://apps.who.int/iris/handle/10665/367620

14. Kim H, Jo MW, Bae SH, Yoon SJ, Lee J. Measuring the burden of disease due to preterm birth complications in Korea using Disability-Adjusted Life Years (DALY). Int J Environ Res Public Health. 2019;16(3):519.

15. World Health Organisation. Diarrhoea [Internet] 2023. Available from: https://www.who.int/health-topics/diarrhoea#tab=tab_1

16. Du Y, Chen C, Zhang X, Yan D, Jiang D, Liu X, et al. Global burden and trends of rotavirus infection-associated deaths from 1990 to 2019: an observational trend study. Virol J. 2022;19(1) Available from: https://virologyj.biomedcentral.com/articles/10.1186/s12985-022-01898-9

17. World Health Organisation. E. coli [Internet]. World Health Organization: WHO; 2018. Available from: https://www.who.int/news-room/fact-sheets/detail/e-coli

18. Disease factsheet about rotavirus [Internet]. European Centre for Disease Prev Control 2017. Available from: https://www.ecdc.europa.eu/en/rotavirus-infection/facts

19. Lazzerini M, Wanzira H. Oral zinc for treating diarrhoea in children. Cochrane Database Syst Rev 2016 (12). Available from: https://www.ncbi.nlm.nih.gov/pmc/articles/PMC5450879/

20. Debellut F, Clark A, Pecenka C, Tate J, Baral R, Sanderson C, Atherly D. Evaluating the potential economic and health impact of rotavirus vaccination in 63 middle-income countries not eligible for Gavi funding: a modelling study. Lancet Global Health. 2021;9(7):942–56. Available from: https://www.thelancet.com/journals/langlo/article/PIIS2214-109X(21)00167-4/fulltext

21. World Health Organisation. Malaria [Internet]. World Health Organization: WHO; 2023. Available from: https://www.who.int/news-room/fact-sheets/detail/malaria
22. Reversing the Incidence of Malaria 2000–2015 [Internet]. 2015. Available from: https://www.unicef.org/media/50711/file/Achieving_the_Malaria_MDG_Target-ENG.pdf
23. World Health Organisation. World malaria report 2022 [Internet]. 2022. Available from: https://www.who.int/publications/i/item/9789240064898
24. 18 million doses of first-ever malaria vaccine allocated to 12 African countries for 2023–2025: Gavi, WHO and UNICEF [Internet] 2023. Available from: https://www.unicef.org/press-releases/18-million-doses-first-ever-malaria-vaccine-allocated-12-african-countries-20232025
25. World Malaria Day: WHO launches effort to stamp out malaria in 25 more countries by 2025 [Internet]. 2021. Available from: https://www.who.int/news/item/21-04-2021-world-malaria-day-who-launches-effort-to-stamp-out-malaria-in-25-more-countries-by-2025
26. World Health Organisation. Malnutrition [Internet]. WHO; 2021. Available from: https://www.who.int/news-room/fact-sheets/detail/malnutrition
27. Victora CG, Christian P, Vidaletti LP, Gatica-Domínguez G, Menon P, Black RE. Revisiting maternal and child undernutrition in low-income and middle-income countries: variable progress towards an unfinished agenda. Lancet. 2021;397(10282) Available from: https://www.thelancet.com/journals/lancet/article/PIIS0140-6736(21)00394-9/fulltext
28. United Nations International Children's Emergency Fund. The State of the World's Children 2019 [Internet]. 2019. Available from: https://www.unicef.org/reports/state-of-worlds-children-2019
29. Black RE, Allen LH, Bhutta ZA, Caulfield LE, de Onis M, Ezzati M, et al. Maternal and child undernutrition: global and regional exposures and health consequences [Internet]. Lancet. 2008;371(9608):243–60. Available from: https://www.thelancet.com/article/S0140-6736(07)61690-0/fulltext
30. World Health Organisation, United Nations International Children's Emergency Fund. Sanitation [Internet]. Available from: https://washdata.org/monitoring/sanitation
31. World Health Organization. Sanitation [Internet]. World Health Organization: WHO; 2022. Available from: https://www.who.int/news-room/fact-sheets/detail/sanitation
32. World Health Organisation, United Nations International Children's Emergency Fund. Progress on household drinking water, sanitation and hygiene 2000–2022: special focus on gender [Internet]. 2023. Available from: https://washdata.org/reports/jmp-2023-wash-households-launch
33. World Health Organisation. SDG Targets 6.1/6.2/6.a Drinking water, sanitation and related official development assistance [Internet]. 2023. Available from: https://www.who.int/data/gho/data/themes/topics/sdg-target-6-ensure-availability-and-sustainable-management-of-water-and-sanitation-for-all
34. World Health Organisation United Nations International Children's Emergency Fund, World Bank. State of the world's drinking water: An urgent call to action to accelerate progress on ensuring safe drinking water for all [Internet]. 2022. Available from: https://www.who.int/publications/i/item/9789240060807
35. Taylor DL, Kahawita TM, Cairncross S, Ensink JHJ. The impact of water, sanitation and hygiene interventions to control cholera: a systematic review. PLOS ONE [Internet]. 2015;10(8) Available from: http://europepmc.org/backend/ptpmcrender.fcgi?accid=PMC4540465&blobtype=pdf
36. Kotloff KL, Riddle MS, Platts-Mills JA, Pavlinac P, Zaidi AKM. Shigellosis. The Lancet. 2018;391(10122):801–12. Available from: https://www.sciencedirect.com/science/article/pii/S0140673617332968
37. World Health Organization. Typhoid [Internet]. World Health Organization: WHO; 2023. Available from: https://www.who.int/news-room/fact-sheets/detail/typhoid

38. Burden of disease attributable to unsafe drinking-water, sanitation and hygiene: 2019 update [Internet]. 2023 June 28. Available from: https://www.who.int/publications/i/item/9789240075610

39. Zdunek K, Blair M, Alexander D. National and public cultures as determinants of health policy and production [Internet]. Issues and Opportunities in Primary Health Care for Children in Europe 2019. Available from: https://www.emerald.com/insight/content/doi/10.1108/978-1-78973-351-820191005/full/html

40. Nyande FK, Ricks E, Williams M, Jardien-Baboo S. Socio-cultural barriers to the delivery and utilisation of child healthcare services in rural Ghana: a qualitative study. BMC Health Serv Res. 2022;22(1):289. Available from: https://bmchealthservres.biomedcentral.com/articles/10.1186/s12913-022-07660-9

41. Azad AD, Charles AG, Ding Q, Trickey AW, Wren SM. The gender gap and healthcare: associations between gender roles and factors affecting healthcare access in Central Malawi, June-August 2017. Arch. Public Health. 2020;78(1):119. Available from: https://archpublichealth.biomedcentral.com/articles/10.1186/s13690-020-00497-w

42. World Health Organization. Regional Office for Europe. Child and adolescent health: fact sheet on Sustainable Development Goals (SDGs): health targets [Internet]. 2017. Available from: https://apps.who.int/iris/handle/10665/340816

43. Sachs J, Schmidt-Traub G, Kroll C, Lafortune G, Fuller G. Sustainable development report 2019. New York: Bertelsmann Stiftung und Sustainable Development Solutions Network (SDSN); 2019. Available at: https://www.bertelsmann-stiftung.de/en/publications/publication/did/sustainable-development-report-2019

44. United Nations The sustainable development goals report 2022 [Internet]. United Nations; 2022. Available from: https://unstats.un.org/sdgs/report/2022/The-Sustainable-Development-Goals-Report-2022.pdf

Chapter 12
Nutrition in Low Resource Countries

Lauren Warrington and Charlotte Wilson

12.1   Definitions of Malnutrition

Malnutrition is defined as 'deficiencies, excesses, or imbalances in a person's intake of energy and/or nutrients' [1]. The term itself therefore encompasses both the 462 million underweight adults and the 1.9 billion overweight or obese adults globally [1]. An individual's dietary requirements are dependent on their age, sex, whether they are pregnant or have a medical condition [2].

Malnutrition describes the three following conditions:

1. Undernutrition

This is described as a **calorie deficiency** resulting in wasting, stunting or underweight individuals that renders them more at risk of disease. Around 45% of deaths among children under 5 years of age are linked to undernutrition [1].

Wasting is due to insufficient food intake or infectious disease. On the other hand, stunting is a result of chronic or recurrent undernutrition which is commonly seen in low socioeconomic status groups.

2. Micro-nutrient related malnutrition

The human body requires a certain daily intake of vitamins and minerals to assist with growth and the production of enzymes and hormones. Micro-nutrient-related malnutrition refers to a deficiency in a specific vitamin or mineral. Key examples of these include iodine, vitamin A and iron.

L. Warrington (✉) · C. Wilson
School of Medicine, Cardiff University, Cardiff, UK
e-mail: lauren.warrington3@wales.nhs.uk; c.wilson73@nhs.net

© The Author(s), under exclusive license to Springer Nature
Switzerland AG 2024
A. Fiander, G. Fry (eds.), *A Healthcare Students Introduction to Global Health*,
https://doi.org/10.1007/978-3-031-66563-9_12

3. Overweight, obesity and diet-related non-communicable diseases

Individuals become overweight when the energy they consume is greater than the energy they expend. This causes abnormal or excessive fat accumulation increasing the risk of non-communicable diseases such as cardiovascular disease. Nowadays, lifestyle changes mean that people are consuming more energy dense foods and drink. They are also partaking in less exercise.

12.2   Underlying Causes of Malnutrition

According to the World Health Organisation (WHO) [1], around 45% of deaths among children under 5 years of age are linked to undernutrition. These deaths mostly occur in low- and middle-income countries where, at the same time, the incidence of childhood obesity is rising.

There are many factors that contribute to malnutrition, but some of the main ones include:

1. *Food environments*

    Food environments are central to the nutritional status of a population. Countries which have increased availability of processed foods and not enough fresh fruit and vegetables are at higher risk of malnutrition [3]. Food environments are determined by both the quality of diet and security of food supply.

    - Quality of diet
      Poor quality diets increase the risk of malnutrition in all its forms. It hinders healthy growth and development. High calorie, low nutritional value diets promote obesity and non-communicable diseases throughout life [3].

    - Food insecurity
      Food insecurity is the disruption of food intake or eating patterns due to a lack of resources. Both undernutrition early in life and childhood obesity increase the risk of non-communicable diseases. This is known as the double burden of malnutrition as it is contributing to global epidemics of long-term conditions such as type 2 diabetes [4].

2. *Physiological factors*

    - Disability
      Physical disability may be associated with reduced mobility, which can hinder a person's ability to access resources, including food. In some cultures, people with disabilities face stigma and discrimination. This can play a role in preventing good nutrition as direct and indirect violence, and maltreatment of people with disabilities means neglect and restricting access to food are accepted in these communities [5].

- Disease
  Prevalence of communicable diseases which cause vomiting and diarrhoea are associated with an increased risk of malnutrition. Non-communicable chronic diseases such as Crohn's disease, among other bowel diseases, affect nutrient absorption and therefore can result in an increased risk of malnutrition [6].

3. *Socio-economic factors*

   - Political and economic situation
     The political and economic situation of a country can have a large effect on a population's nutritional status. For example, war and political unrest can disrupt food supply chains preventing the distribution of food [6].

   - Education
     Educating a population on good nutritional practices such as making healthy food choices and breastfeeding can help reduce the risk of malnutrition [1, 6].

- Poverty
  The main factor that drives contributors of malnutrition is poverty. The inability to afford or access food can be a consequence of many different factors. These can include, but are not limited to:

  - Low status and lack of education for women
  - Insufficient child and maternal care
  - Severe and frequent infections which cause diarrhoea and vomiting
  - War, natural disaster, and civil disorder
  - Unhealthy environments
  - Insufficient household food security

  This demonstrates the multifactorial reality of contributors to malnutrition in a given population. These factors are all interrelated and are underpinned by poverty [6].

12.3   Who Is Most at Risk of Malnutrition?

Malnutrition is not an issue that is exclusive to LRCs; however, it is closely associated with poverty which is known to increase the risks of and from malnutrition. Micronutrient-related malnutrition is more dominant in countries with lower average incomes. Dietary diversity is essential to meeting micronutrient requirements, but poorer households rely on cheaper food commodities such as cereals for energy, and as a result, they lose out on micronutrients.

Women, infants, children and adolescents are each at a particular risk because they have a greater need for nutrients. Adolescent bodies are physically developing in puberty, and without proper nutrition, teenagers can suffer from abnormal development including female menstrual disorders. Infants and children are at the highest risk of dying as they become undernourished faster than adults, are more susceptible to infections and their impaired immune systems prevent quick recovery. Optimising nutrition in the first 1000 days has been argued to be the best solution. However, this cycle all begins with malnourished pregnancies which in turn, place a further generation at risk of the sequential complications of low birth weight [7].

12.4 Micronutrients

Micronutrients are colloquially known as vitamins and minerals. They are not synthesised by the body and therefore must be obtained through diet. Micronutrients are only required in small amounts, but they are essential for healthy development and growth. Deficiencies in micronutrients occur where there is a poor and unvaried diet. Certain population groups, especially women and children, are at greater risk of micronutrient deficiencies [1, 8].

Deficiencies in micronutrients are referred to as hidden hunger and occur when the quality of food people consume does not meet nutritional requirements. It was estimated by United Nations International Children's Emergency Fund (UNICEF) in 2018 that at least 340 million children under 5 suffered from hidden hunger [1].

The WHO [1] identifies iron, vitamin A and iodine as the most important micronutrients in terms of global public health.

IRON Iron is extremely important in healthy cognitive and motor development. A deficiency in iron particularly affects children and pregnant women. Iron deficiency is the leading cause of anaemia which affects 43% of children under 5 years of age and 38% of pregnant women worldwide. This may have severe consequences as it can cause low birth weight in infants and increases the risk of maternal death. Iron and folic acid supplements are both recommended by the WHO to prevent deficiencies in iron [8].

VITAMIN A Vitamin A supports healthy eyesight and enhances immune system function. Children with vitamin A deficiency face an increased risk of blindness and death from infections such as measles and diseases which cause diarrhoea [8].

IODINE Iodine is used by the body to make thyroid hormones. A deficiency in iodine can lead to a spectrum of disorders throughout life, such as hypothyroidism [9]. Iodine is crucial in the early stages of foetal brain development and a deficiency in iodine during pregnancy has been identified as the most significant preventable cause of brain damage [10].

12.5   What Are the Prevention and Treatment Options for Micronutrient Deficiency?

1. *Supplementation*

These are pills, powders or liquid containing high concentrations of micronutrients. Vitamin A supplementation is delivered via high-dose capsules at least twice a year.

2. *Food Fortification*

This option involves processing food frequently consumed by all, adding low concentrations of micronutrients. Iodine deficiency is the leading cause of preventable brain damage in childhood occurring in countries with soils low in iodine content. Universal salt iodisation uses salt to deliver iodine without impacting taste or texture noticeably.

3. *Biofortification and GM crops*

Agronomic and plant-feeding approaches are used to increase the concentration of specific micronutrients in particular crops. A common example is golden rice which is genetically modified to increase beta-carotene content levels; beta-carotene is a vitamin A precursor that that is converted in the body once metabolised. This aims to reduce vitamin A deficiency in LRC to address its health consequences such as blindness and premature death.

12.6   Management

12.6.1   Sustainable Development Goals (SDGs)

Goal 2 of the SDGs of the United Nations (UN) is zero hunger. It calls on all members of the UN to put an end to hunger, achieve food security, improve nutrition and promote sustainable agriculture [11]. A large majority of the 16 other SDGs also work towards promoting and enabling good nutrition. Additionally, the United Nations General Assembly proclaimed a decade of action on nutrition from 2016 to 2025 which further inspired a dedication and commitment worldwide to end hunger whilst also preventing all forms of malnutrition. This increase in global ambition and accountability through the UN has resulted in 163 countries changing their policies and approach to good nutrition [3].

12.6.2   Manuals and Guidelines

Manuals and guidelines help to enable countries to assess the nutritional status of their population. The micronutrient survey manual assesses the micronutrient status of a population and provides information for policy makers and programme implementers to understand the magnitude of micronutrient deficiencies and to collate the information needed to improve programming [12]. Other published guidelines inform policy makers on how to best manage malnutrition within their populations, for example, 'Updates on the management of severe acute malnutrition in infants and children' published by the WHO [13].

12.6.3 Nutrition-Specific

Direct or nutrition-specific approaches address both immediate and underlying causes of malnutrition, such as the treatment of severe acute malnutrition as well as detection of early states of malnutrition. They therefore include interventions in different sectors such as healthcare and education [3].

12.6.4 Nutrition-Sensitive

Nutrition-sensitive approaches to addressing malnutrition differ from nutrition-specific approaches as they are indirect and address more basic and some underlying factors contributing towards malnutrition. They do not target specific nutritional deficiencies but work by improving the chances of an individual accessing a better-quality diet. Examples would be promotion of social safety nets, the empowerment of women and any actions which combat poverty [3].

12.6.5 Systems Approach

It has been found that a systems approach is a better, more holistic way of improving the nutritional status of a population. It combines both nutrition-specific and nutrition-sensitive approaches by drawing on other systems of a society, with five being of particular importance: health, social protection, water and sanitation, education and food systems. It requires a more coordinated approach to help improve and meet nutritional requirements and recognises that the food industry is not a stand-alone sector, encouraging multiple systems to be held accountable for the nutritional status of a population [3].

12.7   What Are the Ethical Considerations for Food Aid?

Food aid refers to the international forms of donating food from one country or institution to another without conventional economic transactions and market mechanisms [14]. This is required to achieve food security globally, but it requires participation from multiple sectors. Below we explore some of the ethical considerations when it comes to food aid:

1. *Access to Food*

Governments and organisations do not have a limitless supply of food aid to meet the demand. They must therefore be discerning in allocating food to where there is the greatest need. There are also logistical considerations involved in this such as means of food distribution.

2. *Food Sovereignty*

To achieve food security, individual or local autonomy and food sovereignty may be ignored so there is the argument whether the right to healthy and culturally acceptable food is more important than the freedom of choice. Exercising individual choice and cultural traditions could also undermine sustainability of food supplies.

3. *Sustainability*

A sustainable diet is one that contains affordable food of adequate nutritional value which leads to better public health, economic stability and has a low impact on the environment. Thus, current cheap labour and cheap raw material are economically and socially unsustainable. This includes wealthier states benefiting off the poverty of LRCs. Sustainability requires action all along the food chain.

4. *Animal Source Foods*

Carnivorous diets are key to the intake of the range of essential micronutrients which plant-based diets struggle to provide in sufficient quantities. However, there is unequal distribution of meat consumption globally with disparities between a country's fraction of the world's population and the percentage of the world's meat they consume. Areas where meat is less frequently eaten is where undernutrition percentage is at its highest such as Africa and South Asia. Fulfilling the nutritional needs of these countries would increase demand for animal source foods, but increased production has negative effects for climate change. Production not only emits a large proportion of greenhouse gases but raises ethical issues around animal welfare. Moreover, maintaining diets rich in animal source foods raises the issue as to whether the one-third of global cereal crop production fed to animals should be redistributed to the starving [15].

5. *Undernutrition vs. Obesity*

LRCs are commonly known to suffer from undernutrition due to governmental failure and poverty, but overweight and obesity are often forgotten about. Obesity is more frequently depicted because of individual choices, yet the causes of all types of malnutrition are linked; a stunted child has an increased risk of being an overweight adult. Therefore, distribution of food aid must look not only at population food intake, but at nutritional value.

12.8   Improving Resilience of Food Supplies

Improving the resilience of food supplies increases the likelihood of them being maintained during unforeseen crises, for example, during war, drought or other natural disasters.

12.8.1   Widening the Range of Suppliers

By increasing the number and range of suppliers, global food systems increase their resilience as they become less reliant on one centralised supply chain. If one supply chain fails, there are more suppliers to cover the deficit ensuring food availability is preserved [16].

12.8.2   Shortening Supply Chains

Shorter supply chains ensure greater resilience in food systems as there are fewer opportunities for error and for links in the chain to be broken. Sourcing food from the local area not only serves as a shorter supply chain but at the same time financially supports local farmers and the local economy [16].

12.8.3   Agroecology

Agroecology describes the application of the study of ecological processes to farming systems. It designs sustainable agroecosystems by applying ecological and agronomic concepts and principles. The term 'agronomic' relates to the application of economic concepts to agricultural systems.

Agroecology is based on sustainable use of natural resources and enhances intrinsic values of ecosystems such as pollination. It encourages the recycling of biomass which reduces the need and demand for expensive and environmentally damaging chemical fertiliser [17]. These systems are more resilient as they have greater capacities to recover from drought, famine, flooding and disease [18]. They encourage diversification of farming practices, so producers have numerous commodities to support themselves if one of the crops or livestock fail [17]. The application of agroecology also shortens the supply chain and reduces dependence on external sources for food supply [18].

12.8.4   Infrastructure

Improvements to infrastructure are important to increase the resilience of food supplies. Examples include building and developing roads to enable easy and efficient transportation of food commodities which additionally makes available an increased number of suppliers. Improving irrigation systems aids with farming and would support and benefit agroeconomic projects [16].

References

1. World Health Organisation. Fact sheets – malnutrition 2020. Available from: https://www.who.int/news-room/fact-sheets/detail/malnutrition
2. World Health Organisation. The double burden of malnutrition 2017. Available from: https://www.who.int/publications/i/item/WHO-NMH-NHD-17.3
3. United Nations International Children's Emergency Fund. The state of the world's children 2019. Available from: https://www.unicef.org/media/60806/file/SOWC-2019.pdf
4. World Health Organisation. More than one in three low- and middle-income countries face both extremes of malnutrition 2019 [12 November 2020]. Available from: https://www.who.int/news/item/16-12-2019-more-than-one-in-three-low%2D%2Dand-middle-income-countries-face-both-extremes-of-malnutrition
5. Rohwerder B. Disability stigma in developing countries. Brighton; 2018. Available from: https://assets.publishing.service.gov.uk/media/5b18fe3240f0b634aec30791/Disability_stigma_in_developing_countries.pdf
6. Müller O, Krawinkel M. Malnutrition and health in developing countries. CMAJ. 2005;173(3):279–86. Available from: https://www.cmaj.ca/content/173/3/279.long
7. Savica. Landscape Report on Adolescent and Maternal Nutrition in Indonesia 2014. Global Alliance for Improved Nutrition (GAIN). Available from: https://www.gainhealth.org/resources/reports-and-publications/landscape-report-adolescent-and-maternal-nutrition-indonesia
8. Centers for Disease Control and Prevention [CDC]. Micronutrient Facts 2020 [12 November 2020]. Available from: https://www.cdc.gov/nutrition/micronutrient-malnutrition/micronutrients/index.html
9. Velasco I, Bath SC, Rayman MP. Iodine as essential nutrient during the first 1000 days of life. Nutrients. 2018;10(3)
10. Toloza FJK, Motahari H, Maraka S. Consequences of severe iodine deficiency in pregnancy: evidence in humans. Front Endocrinol (Lausanne). 2020;11:409.
11. United Nations. Sustainable development goals 2020. Available from: https://sdgs.un.org/goals
12. World Health Organisation. New electronic survey manual supports countries to combat micronutrient deficiencies 2020. Available from: https://www.who.int/news/item/15-10-2020-new-electronic-survey-manual-supports-countries-to-combat-micronutrient-deficiencies
13. World Health Organisation. Guideline: updates on the management of severe acute malnutrition in infants and children Geneva2013. Available from: https://www.who.int/publications/i/item/9789241506328
14. Kortetmäki T. Food aid. In: Kaplan DM, editor. Encyclopedia of food and agricultural ethics. Dordrecht: Springer Netherlands; 2019. p. 958–64.

15. Kortetmäki T. Food security and ethics: the first world hunger. Publisher: Wageningen Academic; 2015. p. 198–204.
16. Béné C. Resilience of local food systems and links to food security—a review of some important concepts in the context of COVID-19 and other shocks. Food Secur. 2020;12(4):805–22.
17. Paracchini M, Wezel A, Madsen S, Stewart B, Karuga J, Attard P, et al. Agroecological practices supporting food production and reducing food insecurity in developing countries—a study on scientific literature in 17 countries. Luxembourg; 2020.
18. Food and Agriculture Organisation of the United Nations. The 10 elements of agroecology 2020. Available from: https://www.fao.org/agroecology/overview/overview10elements/en/

Chapter 13
Mental Health in Low Resource Countries

Chantal Corbin and Jasmin Johnson

13.1 Introduction

Mental Health: Definition
Mental health is defined as 'a state of well-being in which every individual realizes his or her own potential, can cope with the normal stresses of life, can work productively and fruitfully, and is able to make a contribution to her or his community' (WHO).

The term 'mental health' is often used interchangeably with 'mental illness'; however, the two are distinct. Mental illness refers to any health condition affecting a person's behaviour and emotions and, if severe, results in functional impairment and interference in daily activities [1].

Although approximately 80% of the global population live in low- and middle-income countries (LMICs), research and data exploring mental health in these countries are scarce. In fact, only 6% of the available data comes from these countries [2].

An understanding of the burden of mental health disease in low resource countries (LRCs) and proposed policy implications to better manage mental health in these countries will be explored in this chapter. Tackling this burden not only ensures that the goal of Universal Health Coverage declared by the World Health

C. Corbin (✉)
School of Medicine, Cardiff University, Cardiff, UK
e-mail: corbincr@cardiff.ac.uk

J. Johnson
Cardiff University, Cardiff, UK
e-mail: johnsonj28@cardiff.ac.uk

© The Author(s), under exclusive license to Springer Nature Switzerland AG 2024
A. Fiander, G. Fry (eds.), *A Healthcare Students Introduction to Global Health*, https://doi.org/10.1007/978-3-031-66563-9_13

Organisation (WHO) is closer to being accomplished, but on an individual basis, like any other successfully treated disease, will increase a person's healthy life years.

13.2   The Burden of Mental Health Disorders in Low Resource Countries

Mental health disorders (MHDs) encompass mood, anxiety and personality, along with neurological and substance abuse-related disorders. It is thought that one in eight people is affected by a mental health disorder. Globally, this equates to 970 million people at one time experiencing poor mental health [3]; this is greater than the entire population of Europe.

MHDs are the leading culprit of people living with morbidity worldwide. It is estimated that MHDs are responsible for 16% of disability-adjusted life years (DALYs) [4].

> **Global Burden of Disease for Mental Health Disorders**
> The global burden of mental health disease is underestimated. Vigo et al. estimate that mental health disorders globally account for 32.4% of the years lived with disability (YLDs) and 13% of the global disability-adjusted life years (DALYs). This places the global burden of disease which can be attributed to MHD level with that of cardiovascular disease in terms of DALYs [5].

MHDs affect every country and community over the world; however in LRCs, MHDs often go undiagnosed and untreated. In LRCs, plagued by violence and conflict due to war or civil unrest, the number of people suffering from mental ill health increases from the global average of 10 to 22.1%. This is the equivalent of approximately one in five people [6].

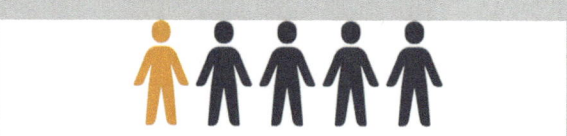
Global average prevalence of MHD increases from 10% to 22.1% in LRCs.

Global average prevalence of MHD increases from 10% to 22.1% in LRCs

Equating to 1 in 5 People [6]

Despite the heavily weighted burden of disease, in LRCs, it is estimated that 75% of people do not have access to the mental health support they require. This is, in part, attributed to the number of mental health professionals working in LRCs, which is as low as 2 per 100,000 people in some communities. This is quite clearly insufficient as 1 in 10 people will require mental health support or treatment at any one time [7].

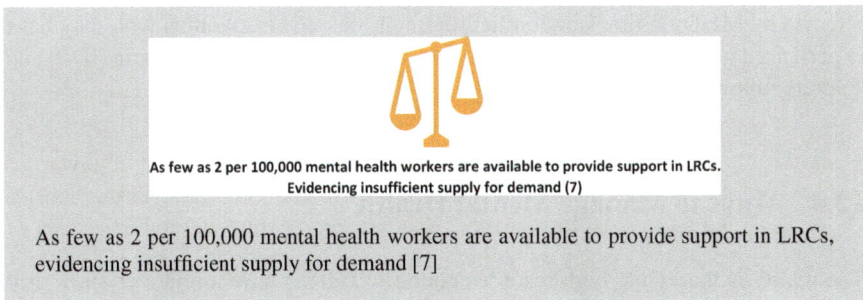

As few as 2 per 100,000 mental health workers are available to provide support in LRCs, evidencing insufficient supply for demand [7]

In LRCs, MHDs account for 9.8% of the total burden of disease, which increases to 11.1% with the addition of injuries which are self-inflicted, i.e. self-harm and suicide. Depression, specifically unipolar depressive disorder, is the leading neuropsychiatric cause of burden of disease [2].

Unipolar depressive disorder is the leading cause of burden of disease [2].

Disorders of mental health are chronic and debilitating. Mental health conditions decrease productivity and have an enormous impact on family and friends. MHDs are also known to be a major risk factor for various other health conditions. Take, for example, the secondary effects of alcohol abuse such as liver disease and ischaemic heart disease. The co-morbidities threaten to further impair and possibly shorten the life of those affected.

Sadly, severe mental health disorders contribute to the global burden of suicide. Globally, the WHO estimates that 800,000 people die because of suicide each year. In low resource countries, 1.5% of all deaths are a result of self-inflicted injuries [7, 8].

It is important to remember that the disease burden of mental disorders has estimated values. There is likely to be considerable underreporting and so underestimation, due to stigma and cultural perceptions of MHDs and events such as suicide. Furthermore, lack of education and the ability to accurately diagnose MHD pose further barriers to the reporting of the burden of disease.

13.3 Social Determinants of Mental Health Disorders in Low Resource Countries

Many parallels can be drawn between the state of mental health in HRCs and LRCs. However, some exacerbating factors are more frequently or more severely experienced in LRCs such as humanitarian crises including natural disasters, war and displacement. These events have hugely deleterious consequences on the mental health of the population. Subsets of the population in LRCs are disproportionately affected by MHD; in times of conflict, these groups include women who may have experienced gender-based violence, refugees, internally displaced people (IDP) and soldiers following war.

13.4 Ways to Manage Mental Health

The reality is that while high resource countries (HRC) have a relatively firm grip on the burden of mental illness through pharmacological, psychoeducation and social treatments, which have proven effective, these cannot be easily transferred to LRCs, which differ socially, culturally and economically.

At the core, managing mental health first requires the uprooting of deeply embedded cultural stigma and illiteracy on mental disorders. Without this mindset shift, little change can be made. Though charities and humanitarian outreach programmes exist which dedicate their time and resources to LRCs, this is a mere sticking plaster, rather governments must look to a sustainable resolution which originates within the country itself.

13.5 So, How Can We Better Manage Mental Health in LRCs?

13.5.1 Address Mental Health Illiteracy and Stigma

In many LRCs, particularly India and African countries, stigma around mental illness is deeply embedded in the culture, with a view that people are possessed by demons and cursed [9, 10]. Hence, many are shunned from their families and society at large and are not provided with the care they need. Individuals can often resort to suicide as a result.

> When it is spiritual, doctors can do all they have learnt from books, it will never work.
> (Prophet Kweku Nii Okai, 2018)

Education in schools and communities is a crucial step in raising awareness about mental health and educating on appropriate coping mechanisms. This is effective when delivered in small village groups, led by a trusted volunteer who can instigate meaningful dialogue. Public health campaigns can also play a role, employing colloquial language to convey important messages about mental health. Finally, celebrities and influential figures are able to use their platform to dismantle misconceptions surrounding the topic. Many celebrities have begun to do this, sharing their own personal stories which are likely to resonate in particular with young people.

De-stigmatisation of mental illness will inevitably lead to an increase in persons seeking relevant care to improve their quality of life.

13.5.2 Investment in Mental Health

13.5.2.1 Redistribution of Monetary Resources

Currently, LRCs such as countries in Africa and South-East Asia allocate less than 1% of their healthcare budget to mental health [2]. The funding that is available is directed towards affluent areas and psychiatric hospitals for patients with severe mental health disorders. This contradicts the efforts being made by the World Health Organisation (WHO) for universal health coverage for all. Irrespective of the severity of a mental health disorder, individuals should be offered equal access to effective and affordable care. An audit could be undertaken to identify superfluous areas of spending within national and healthcare budgets and redistribute excess funds accordingly.

13.5.2.2 Incremental Increase of the Mental Health Budget

Some LRCs currently spend $0.20 per person per annum (pppa) on mental health. This is well below the suggested $2 pppa [11]. Understandably, governments may not be in the financial position to augment their budget with immediate effect. However, an incremental approach should be considered. It is estimated that allocating $1 pppa for depressive and bipolar disorders covers 33% of the affected population; this increases to 50% coverage when $2 pppa is allocated.

13.5.2.3 Prevalence Assessments

The mental health burdens and healthcare systems vary within LRCs; therefore, it is important to not apply a one-size-fits-all approach to mental health budget allocation and generalised solutions. Instead, individual countries need to undertake occasional audits aimed at assessing the burden of disease, the population's needs and available services. This information is crucial in preventing under- and over-budgeting within a particular sector of mental health.

Upon provision of adequate funding for a mental health budget, practical applications to manage the disease burden can be sought.

The Alma-Ata Declaration of 1978 highlighted the key role that primary health-care has in universal healthcare. This action is relevant in LRCs especially where studies suggest that primary healthcare should be more involved in the management of mental health conditions, given that patients generally tend to present within this setting. However, involvement of primary health professionals can only lessen the burden on the healthcare system to a certain extent. As such, it has been suggested that a step-up care model is adopted [2, 11].

This involves the training of lay people in villages to assess, counsel and where necessary, refer mental health patients. In Africa, traditional medical practitioners are reputable and highly influential in the community (Fig. 13.1).

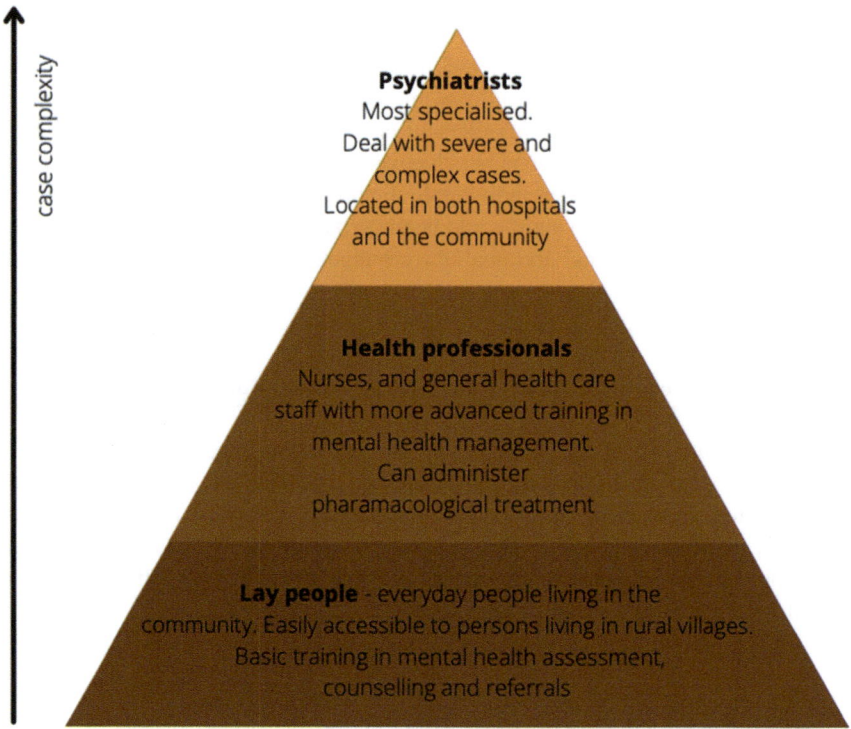

Fig. 13.1 Pyramid showing the pyramidal approach to mental healthcare. The implementation of trained lay people allows a larger proportion of the population to have access to care irrespective of the remoteness of villages [11]

13.6 Managing Mental Health Through Prioritisation of an Adequate Mental Health Budget

This is based on the understanding that a social and cultural mindset shift must first occur (Fig. 13.2).

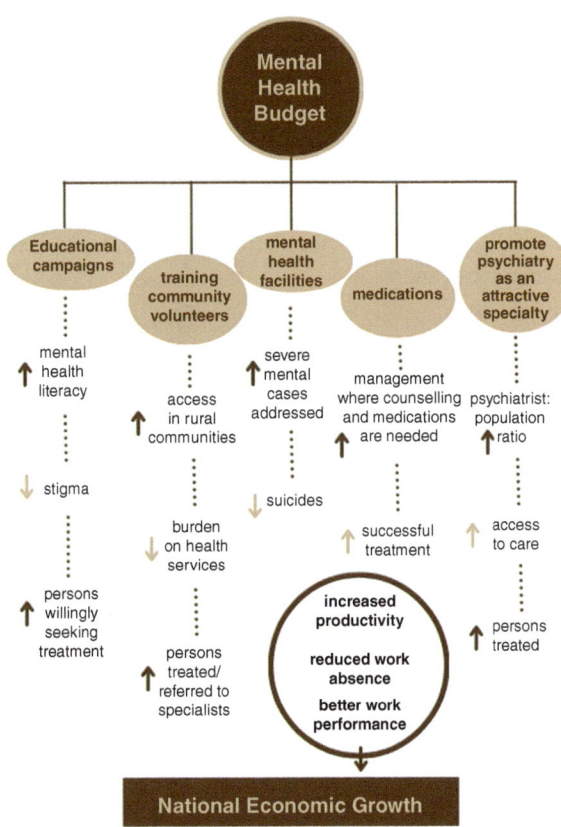

Fig. 13.2 A diagram illustrating ways in which an adequate mental health budget can be apportioned with the aim of reducing the burden of mental health disease in low resource countries. This involves targeting culturally embedded stigma, recruiting and training of mental health volunteers, increasing the number of specialty facilities, sourcing medications and promoting psychiatry as a specialty. It also highlights the theoretical economic return resulting from investment in the mental health of the population

13.7   Conclusion

Generally, mental health in LRCs is underfunded and overlooked. However, the burden of disease cannot be ignored; mental health disorders account for the greatest cause of years lived with a disability, with the impact on individuals being severe and long lasting. As with all countries, socioeconomic status is dependent upon the ability of a population to thrive.

Evidently, funding is required to improve mental health provision in LRCs. Adequate mental health service provision is a necessity; however, for this to be implemented, local professionals must undergo mental health training. Simultaneously, education during childhood and adolescence about mental health is paramount to the destigmatisation of mental health disorders currently prevalent in many cultures.

With mental health awareness increasing globally, it is anticipated that LRCs will follow suit and devise actionable strategies to tackle mental health within their respective borders.

References

1. What is mental illness? In: Psychiatry.org—what is mental illness? https://www.psychiatry.org/patients-families/what-is-mental-illness. Accessed 21 Apr 2021.
2. Patel V. Mental health in low- and middle-income countries. Br Med Bull. 2007;81–82:81–96.
3. Global Health Data Exchange (GHDx). In: Institute for Health Metrics and Evaluation. https://vizhub.healthdata.org/gbd-results/. Accessed 21 Apr 2021.
4. Arias D, Saxena S, Verguet S. Quantifying the global burden of mental disorders and their economic value. eClinicalMedicine. 2022;54:101675.
5. Vigo D, Thornicroft G, Atun R. Estimating the true global burden of mental illness. Lancet Psychiatry. 2016;3:171–8.
6. The World Bank: Mental Health. https://www.worldbank.org/en/topic/mental-health. Accessed 21 Apr 2021.
7. Mental health atlas 2020. In: World Health Organization. https://www.who.int/publications-detail-redirect/9789240036703. Accessed 21 Apr 2021.
8. 1. (1970) Suicide in the world: global health estimates. In: World Health Organization. https://apps.who.int/iris/handle/10665/326948. Accessed 21 Apr 2021.
9. (2018) Caged while seeking mental health help—BBC News, YouTube. Available at: https://www.youtube.com/watch?v=p9Pl0MGu2YQ
10. (2015) Locked up and forgotten: India's mental health crisis. YouTube Available at: https://www.youtube.com/watch?v=Ux14_DEw7Hs
11. Mackenzie J, Caddick H. How low-income countries can invest in mental health—ODI https://cdn.odi.org/media/documents/11183.pdf. Accessed 21 Apr 2021.

Chapter 14
Road Traffic Accidents in Low-Resource Countries

Mariam Al-Ani

14.1 Who RTAs Affect

- In 2019, road traffic accidents were ranked as the sixth top global cause of disability-adjusted life years (DALYs) by the World Health Organisation (WHO) [1].
- Each year, more than 1.3 million people lose their lives in road traffic accidents, and those mainly affected are vulnerable road users such as pedestrians, cyclists and motorcyclists.
- Road traffic accidents are the main cause of death in children and young adults.
- Low- and middle-resource countries are where 93% of fatalities occur, despite having only 60% of the world's vehicles.
- Young males are three times more likely to be killed in a road traffic accident than young females [2].

14.2 Risk Factors for RTAs

1. SPEEDING. Speeding increases both the probability of a crash occurring and the severity of the injury. A 1% increase in speed causes a 4% increase in the risk of a fatal crash [2]. A study found that half of the reported crashes in Ghana between 1998 and 2000 were due to the 'speed factor' alone [3].
2. ALCOHOL/SUBSTANCES. Driving under the influence of substances or alcohol increases the risk of a car crash. In a hospital survey in Kenya, 40% of

M. Al-Ani (✉)
School of Medicine, Cardiff University, Cardiff, UK

137

patients undergoing post-crash treatment were under the influence of alcohol at the time of the crash [4].

3. NOT USING HELMETS, SEAT BELTS and CHILD RESTRAINTS. This leads to a higher risk of death and disability. Many countries do not have mandatory requirements, and if they do, they are not often enforced [5].

4. DISTRACTIONS. Distractions include mobile phone use, eating or drinking, smoking, adjusting car controls or talking to passengers [6].

5. UNSAFE ROADS. Roads are often poorly designed, not maintained and frequently contain a blend of road users [7]. A study in Ghana revealed that 41% of fatal casualties from crashes were among pedestrian road users and rear-end collisions [8].

6. UNSAFE VEHICLES. Only 40 countries in the world meet all the UN vehicle safety standards regulations, which includes seat belts, frontal and side impact protection, pedestrian protection, child restraints and electronic stability control [7].

7. INADEQUATE LAW ENFORCEMENT. Many countries do have laws addressing the use of seat belts, drink-driving and speeding; however, they are not adequately enforced due to limited financial and human resources, corruption and lack of political will [7].

14.3 Challenges for Treating RTAs

– After a crash has occurred, there are multiple barriers for patients to access medical care:

14.3.1 Pre-hospital Care

1. Availability of appropriate infrastructure. There is often poor coordination and a lack of a trauma system in LRCs [2]. Patients are often collected and transported by a passer-by which increases the risk of secondary injuries [9].

2. Traffic congestion. The consequences of road traffic outcomes are time-sensitive, and delays caused by poor road infrastructure and traffic jams lead to the late arrival of emergency services and a high incidence of secondary crashes and injuries [10]. In a study in India, 58% of patients who died did so at the scene of the crash and 7% on the way to the hospital [11].

14.3.2 Hospital Care

3. Medical treatment. Lack of emergency medical services combined with a lack of physicians, surgeons and anaesthetists lead to worse outcomes in LRCs [12].

4. Rehabilitation. All patients with severe injury and half of the patients with moderate injury require long-term rehabilitation. This requires MDT input with physiotherapy, occupational therapy, time off work and rest. In LRCs, these are not widely available [11].

14.3.3   Consequences

– Economic burden. Road traffic injuries carry a high cost; one study estimates that the global cost of RTAs was $518 billion US dollars [13].
– Societal burden. It is hard to measure the exact societal burden, as road traffic injuries and mortalities have long-standing and far-reaching effects. In LRCs, good free medical care and rehabilitation is scarce, and so patient care often relies heavily on the patient, their friends and their family to carry the financial burden and physical and psychological stress [14].
– Psychological burden. There is also a significant long-term psychological burden associated with depression and post-traumatic stress disorder [14].

14.3.4   Prevention

– Road traffic accidents are predictable and preventable, and many strategies exist to reduce the numbers and consequences associated.
    5. ROAD USER. This involves education about safe driving, enforcing speed limits and checking blood alcohol concentrations. Helmet wearing reduces death risk by 40%, and in Vietnam in 2007, the motorcycle helmet policy increased the use of helmets from 30% to 93%. This prevented approximately 2200 deaths and 29,000 head injuries, saving over US $18 million [15]. Seat belt use reduces deaths by 50%, and child use restraint reduces the likelihood of injury for children by up to 80% [16].
    6. VEHICLE. Increasing vehicle safety technology decreases the fatality of a car crash. In LRCs, these vehicles are scarce and costly and require enforcement of vehicle safety standards [7].
    7. INFRASTRUCTURE. This includes separating pedestrians and motorists, adequate lighting, lane markings, roadside barriers and pedestrian crossings. Other measures include speed bumps or rumble strips [14].

– In 2017, the WHO produced a technical road safety package with a 'Save LIVES' approach [7]. It contains 6 effective strategies and 22 interventions which are summarised with the following acronym:
    • S (save)—Speed management.
    • L—Leadership in road safety.

- • I—Infrastructure and design improvement.
- • V—Vehicle safety standards.
- • E—Enforcement of traffic laws.
- • S—Survival after a crash.

- There are challenges in implementing these strategies, including economic, and cultural beliefs, and low literacy rates [17].

14.4   Summary

Road traffic accidents represent a large global burden of disease with vast consequences particularly affecting low-resource countries. However, RTAs are predictable and preventable and require increased legislation of road safety policy to reduce mortality and morbidity.

References

1. World Health Organization. Life expectancy and leading causes of death and disability. Switzerland: WHO's Global Health Estimates Internet. Available from: https://www.who.int/data/gho/data/themes/mortality-and-global-health-estimates [Google Scholar] (2019).
2. World Health Organisation: Road traffic injuries. https://www.who.int/news-room/fact-sheets/detail/road-traffic-injuries (2021). Accessed 13 Apr 2022.
3. Afukaar FK. Speed control in developing countries: issues, challenges and opportunities in reducing road traffic injuries. Inj Control Saf Promot. 2003;10(1–2):77–81. https://doi.org/10.1076/icsp.10.1.77.14113.
4. Odero W, Khayesi M, Heda PM. Road traffic injuries in Kenya: magnitude, causes and status of intervention. Inj Control Saf Promot. 2003;10(1–2):53–61. https://doi.org/10.1076/icsp.10.1.53.14103.
5. Road Traffic Injuries Research Network Multicenter Study C, Williams A, Francis A, Williams A, Trinh Thuy A, Hejar AR, et al. The use of non-standard motorcycle helmets in low- and middle-income countries: a multicentre study. Inj Prev. 2013;19(3):158. https://doi.org/10.1136/injuryprev-2012-040348.
6. World Health Organization, NHTSA. Mobile phone use: a growing problem of driver distraction. Geneva: World Health Organization; 2011.
7. World Health Organization. Save LIVES —a road safety technical package 2017.
8. Damsere-Derry J, Palk G, King M. Road accident fatality risks for "vulnerable" versus "protected" road users in northern Ghana. Traffic Inj Prev. 2017;18(7):736–43. https://doi.org/10.1080/15389588.2017.1302083.
9. Moore L, Champion H, Tardif P-A, Kuimi B-L, O'Reilly G, Leppaniemi A, et al. Impact of trauma system structure on injury outcomes: a systematic review and meta-analysis. World J Surg. 2018;42(5):1327–39. https://doi.org/10.1007/s00268-017-4292-0.
10. Khorasani-Zavareh D, Khankeh HR, Mohammadi R, Laflamme L, Bikmoradi A, Haglund BJA. Post-crash management of road traffic injury victims in Iran. Stakeholders' views on current barriers and potential facilitators. BMC Emerg Med. 2009;9(1):8. https://doi.org/10.1186/1471-227X-9-8.

11. Hsiao M, Malhotra A, Thakur JS, et al. Road traffic injury mortality and its mechanisms in India: nationally representative mortality survey of 1.1 million homes. BMJ Open. 2013;3:e002621. https://doi.org/10.1136/bmjopen-2013-002621.
12. Hung Y-C, Bababekov YJ, Stapleton SM, Mukhopadhyay S, Huang S-L, Briggs SM, et al. Reducing road traffic deaths: where should we focus global health initiatives? J Surg Res. 2018;229:337–44. https://doi.org/10.1016/j.jss.2018.04.036.
13. Jacobs G, Aeron-Thomas A, Astrop A. Estimating global road fatalities. TRL report no 445. Crowthorne: Transport Research Laboratory. 2000.
14. Bachani AM, Peden M, Gururaj G, Norton R, Hyder AA. Road traffic injuries. In: Mock CN, Nugent R, Kobusingye O, Smith KR, editors. Injury prevention and environmental health. Washington, DC: The International Bank for Reconstruction and Development/The World Bank. 2017. © 2017 International Bank for Reconstruction and Development/The World Bank.
15. Olson Z, Staples JA, Mock C, Nguyen NP, Bachani AM, Nugent R, et al. Helmet regulation in Vietnam: impact on health, equity and medical impoverishment. Inj Prev. 2016;22(4):233. https://doi.org/10.1136/injuryprev-2015-041650.
16. Zaloshnja E, Miller TR, Hendrie D. Effectiveness of child safety seats vs safety belts for children aged 2 to 3 years. Arch Pediatr Adolesc Med. 2007;161(1):65. https://doi.org/10.1001/archpedi.161.1.65.
17. Forjuoh SN. Traffic-related injury prevention interventions for low-income countries. Inj Control Saf Promot. 2003;10(1–2):109–18. https://doi.org/10.1076/icsp.10.1.109.14115.

Chapter 15
Burns in Low Resource Countries

Ishak Abdikadir Mohamed

15.1 Burns and Their Significance in LRCs

- The World Health Organisation (WHO) defines a burn as an 'injury to the skin or other organic tissue primarily caused by heat or due to radiation, radioactivity, electricity, friction or contact with chemicals' [1].
- Non-fatal burn injuries are the leading cause of morbidity; however, they are frequently preventable.
- There are an estimated 180,000 deaths annually as a direct consequence of burns, with a large proportion of these deaths occurring in LRCs.
- Health losses because of burns come in different forms, from lifelong disability to death in extreme cases.

15.2 Key Statistics Relating to Childhood Burns

- Worldwide, the burden of child burn deaths is 2.5 per 100,000 across 103 countries with the largest burden in Sub-Saharan Africa [2].
- In 2018, mortality rates from burns in children were over 7 times higher in low- and middle-income countries than in higher-income countries [1]. This huge disparity in mortality rates highlights the gravity of the issue in LRCs.
- For example, in a lower-middle income country like Bangladesh, nearly 173,000 children are moderately or severely burned every year.

I. A. Mohamed (✉)
School of Medicine, Cardiff University, Cardiff, UK

15.3 Causes of Burns

- Most burns in LRCs occur in the home, where open flames are frequently used for cooking and warmth, explaining the annual peak in burns in some African regions during the cold Harmattan season from November to February [3]. See Figs. 15.1 and 15.2.
- Furthermore, women aged between 16 and 35 are recognised to be the most susceptible to burns within households. This is a direct consequence of their predominant roles in cooking for the family unit. Their loose clothing also contributes further to their increased risk of burns [4].

Summary of findings by studies on special cases of burn injuries

Type of Injury	Critical Findings
Stove Burns	• Women 20-29 years of age are the most of risk • Most are of low SES • Injuries most often occur during cooking or refilling
Bed Net Burns	• Most individuals are one year of age or less • Most are male • Most suffer > 20 % TBSA
Intentional and Unintentional Chemical burns	• Chemical assault are often suffered by males and are a result of acid thrown at the face, head and neck • Chemical ingestion are most often acids if accidental and alkalis if intentional • Of cases of ingestions, most individuals are of low SES
Intentional Burns	• Many are suffered by females 20-30 years of age using flame in a suicide attempt • Assaults of men by their partners are also described, often by hot liquids • Many are a results of relationship difficulties
Electrical Burns	• Most of those injured are male • Most are between 20-40 years of age • The extremities are most commonly affected
Occupational Burns	• Most are males • Most suffer approximately 20% TBSA • Most injuries are flame burns

SES, socio-economic status ; TBSA, total body surface area

Fig. 15.1 Types of burns [4]

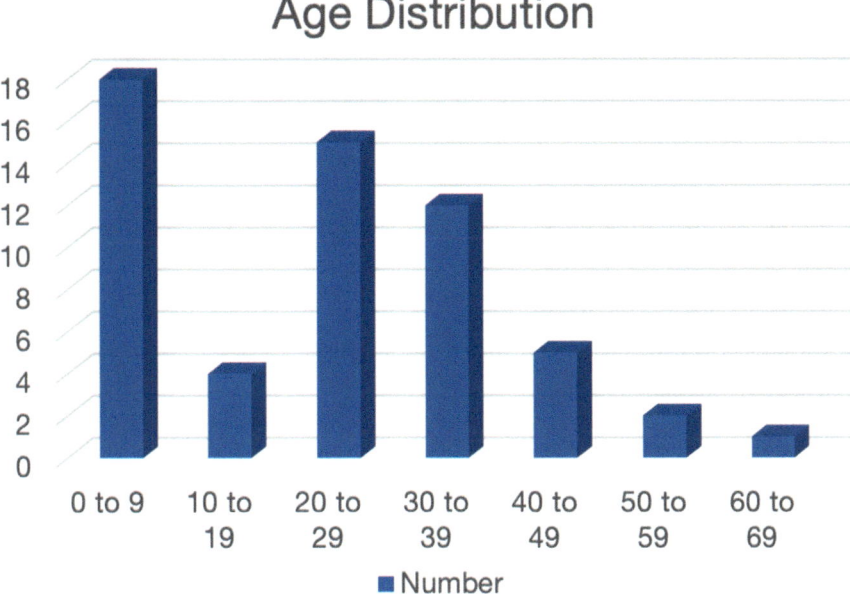

Fig. 15.2 Diagram showing the age distribution of burn patients in a hospital in Lagos, Nigeria [5]

- In terms of epidemiological factors of paediatric burns, the most common cause of burns in children is their relative access to home appliances. Further emphasis needs to therefore be placed on the supervision of children given that unsupervised children are at higher risk of burn-related injury.
- According to the African Journal of Emergency Medicine, reports of scalds in the upper extremities are the most common types of burn injuries in children [4, 5].
- It is important to note that a small proportion of burns in LRCs are also caused by underlying medical conditions, including epilepsy, peripheral neuropathy, and physical and cognitive disabilities. This is coupled with inadequate safety measures for liquefied petroleum gas and electricity [1].

15.4 Consequences of Burns

Damage from burns has consequences on the affected individual, their family and society at large. The direct consequences of burns can be categorised into three main groups:

15.4.1 Medical

Burns can cause severe medical complications depending on the scale of the burn and the site of the burn on the human body (see Fig. 15.3).

- Relative age of the patient has a correlation with the types of burns suffered and the degree of the burn.
- Children suffer from more severe burns because their skin is breached more easily [6].
- The most common anatomical position of burns is in the upper limbs, with 83% of the patients admitted suffering such burns.
- Over 65% of patients admitted had their trunk affected as a result of burns in the head and neck region [5].
- Burns where the head and trunk are affected will result in other serious complications such as a blocked airway, which may require surgical intervention.
- Wound infection is the most common early complications in the acute phase.
- Pneumonia and septicaemia were also the common early acute complications in patients suffering from burns and scalds.

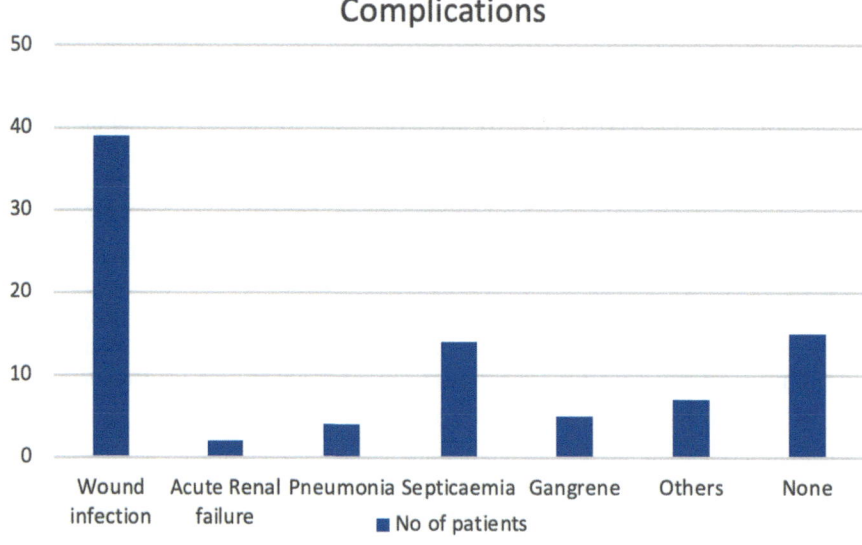

Fig. 15.3 Diagram showing the early complications of wounds in a hospital in Lagos, Nigeria [5]

15.4.2   Economic

15.4.2.1   Case Study: Kamuzu Central Hospital Burn Unit in Lilongwe, Malawi [7]

Gallaher et al. [7] state that burn care in LRCs is very 'dependent on the availability of financial resources, equipment and expertise' (Fig. 15.4)

- In essence, where there is lack of funding, resources or expertise, there will naturally be a decline in the quality of burn care that is provided (Fig. 15.5).
- The largest cost component in acute burn cases is wound dressings
- Whilst the costs of surgery, clinic visits and physiotherapy are not that high, these would all be required for more severe complications of burns, therefore highlighting the main problems faced by LRC, where lack of funding hinders the treatment of serious complications.

15.4.3   Social

The social factors of burn-related trauma influence the LRC's economy.

- Burns and scar formation can be damaging for the individual and how they approach their daily lives.

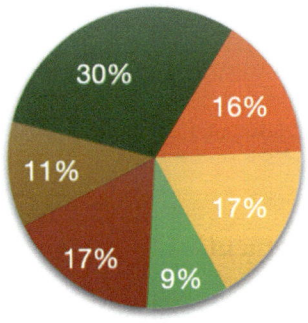

Total Monthly burns

- Clinical Consumables   ($1,803.63)   ■ Medications   ($2,030.41)
- Ancillary   ($1,503.24)   ■ Human Resources   ($1,928.00)
- Operative Cost   ($1,325.88)   ■ Facility Cost   ($3,481.50)

Fig. 15.4 Graph showing the percentage composition of total monthly burn expenditures in Kamuzu Central Hospital, Malawi [7]

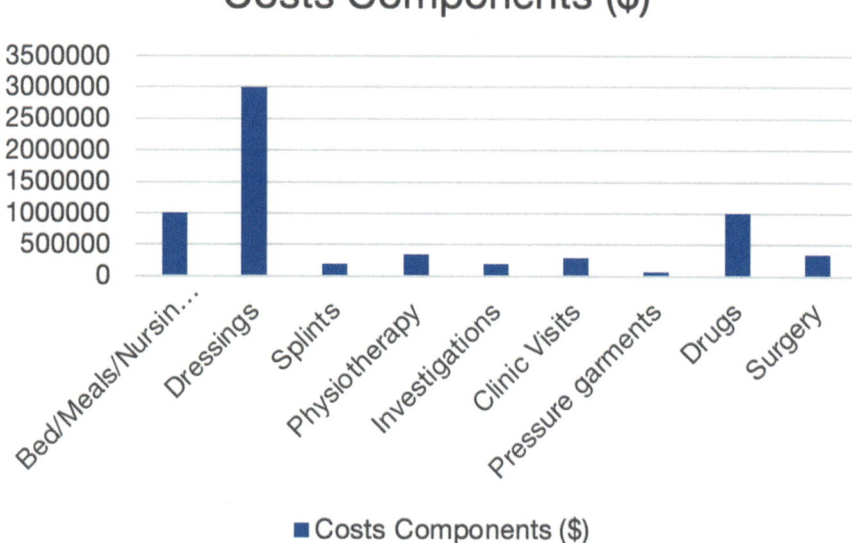

Fig. 15.5 Diagram showing the distribution pattern of the costs of management of acute burns in a hospital in Lagos, Nigeria [5]

- Lack of surgical or medical intervention in most cases will result in disabilities or having to take time off work.
- From a social perspective, this can have profound impact on the affected individual.
- Their lives can be permanently altered, as well as their physical appearance.
- Having to take time off work has grave consequences in low-income households, especially in LRCs.
- Males constitute 90% of work-related burns—in some cases where the burns are severe, this raises a dilemma if the male in a household is the only source of income or the main breadwinner.

15.5 Burns Management

The acute management of burns essentially depends on the anatomical position of the burn and the subsequent degree of the burn. The National Institute of Health and Care Excellence (NICE) recommends that the appropriate management of wounds in primary care should involve wound cleaning, debridement, blister management, wound dressing and reassessment. However, hospital admission may be required for more severe wounds [6].

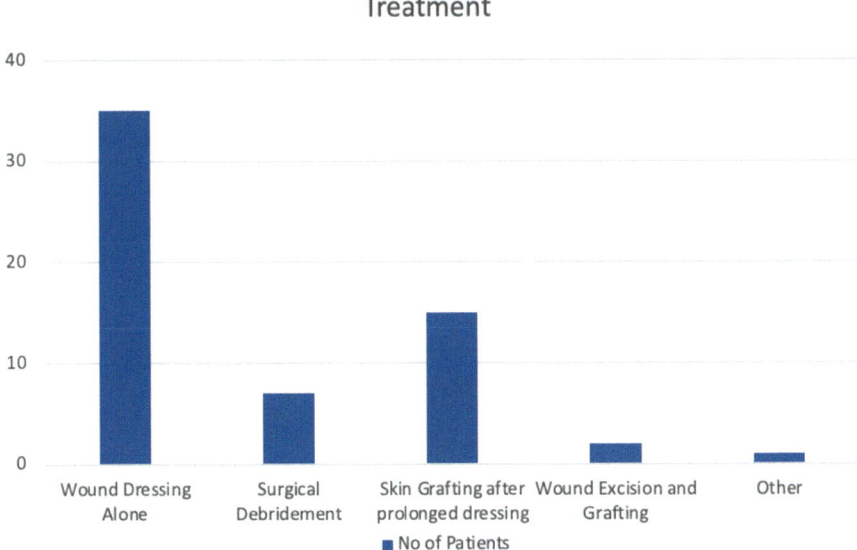

Fig. 15.6 Diagram showing the different methods of treatment of burn cases in a hospital in Lagos, Nigeria [5]

Figure 15.6 illustrates the mode of treatment and management of patients who presented with burns and scalds with the initial presentation of the symptoms from a low-resource country in sub-Saharan Africa.

- Most patients undergo treatment using wound dressings alone.
- This is significant, as whilst the wound dressing application is integral in the prevention of infections and disease, the word 'alone' highlights the lack of other medical interventions for patients with second- or third-degree burns.

15.5.1 Challenges in Burns Treatment

- Most hospitals in LRCs are ill-equipped for burn management.
- Operating theatres in LRCs may have poor physical facilities.
- There are insufficient numbers of staff trained in burns management in LRCs.
- LRCs have a much lower doctor to patient ratio.

Lack of access to safe, affordable and timely surgical care and anaesthesia continues to be a major global health problem, and one that is affecting the delivery of appropriate burn care, with an estimated 5 billion people worldwide currently without access to this kind of care. [8]

15.6 Burn Prevention Methods

See Ref. [1]

- Improving awareness of risk factors which cause burns such as loose clothing and open wood fires
- Teaching and training in basic first aid
- Funding the development of houses with better cooking facilities—remove cooking pots at ground level
- Deliver burn prevention programmes

15.6.1 Challenges in Burn Prevention

Many health agencies, corporations' authorities and even medical personnel in LRCs prioritise disease prevention over injury prevention [9]:

- Injury prevention policies are absent in LRCs, and therefore, burns prevention programmes have failed to receive required government funding.
- Moreover, lack of government initiative and limited access to media in most LRCs preclude effective prevention programmes [9].
- In the USA, the average cost of providing satisfactory care for a patient with burn injuries is approximately US$1000, which is not feasible in an LRC.

References

1. World Health Organization. Burns 2018. Available from: https://www.who.int/news-room/fact-sheets/detail/burns
2. Sengoelge M, El-Khatib Z, Laflamme L. The global burden of child burn injuries in light of country level economic development and income inequality. Prev Med Rep. 2017;6:115–20.
3. Thomson IK, Iverson KR, Innocent SHS, Kaseje N, Johnson WD. Management of paediatric burns in low- and middle-income countries: assessing capacity using the World Health Organization Surgical Assessment Tool. Int Health. 2020;12(5):499–506.
4. Rybarczyk MM, Schafer JM, Elm CM, Sarvepalli S, Vaswani PA, Balhara KS, et al. A systematic review of burn injuries in low- and middle-income countries: epidemiology in the WHO-defined African region. Afr J Emerg Med. 2017;7(1):30–7.
5. Ahachi CN, Fadeyibi IO, Abikoye FO, Chira MK, Ugburo AO, Ademiluyi SA. The direct hospitalization cost of care for acute burns in Lagos, Nigeria: a one-year prospective study. Ann Burns Fire Disasters. 2011;24(2):94–101.
6. National Institute for health and care excellence. Burns and scalds 2020. Available from: https://cks.nice.org.uk/topics/burns-scalds/
7. Gallaher JR, Mjuweni S, Cairns BA, Charles AG. Burn care delivery in a sub-Saharan African unit: a cost analysis study. Int J Surg. 2015;19:116–20.
8. Stokes MAR, Johnson WD. Burns in the third world: an unmet need. Ann Burns Fire Disasters. 2017;30(4):243–6.
9. Atiyeh B, Masellis A, Conte F. Optimizing burn treatment in developing low-and middle-income countries with limited health care resources (part 3). Ann Burns Fire Disasters. 2010;23(1):13–8.

Chapter 16
Cancer in Low- and Middle-Income Countries

Upha Barclay, Olivia Curtis-Hughes, Molly Evans, and Hannah Raval

16.1 What Is the Epidemiology of Cancer?

Cancer contributes to a significant burden of disease in low- and middle-income countries (LMICs). Globally, cancers, grouped together, are the second greatest cause of death, following cardiovascular diseases [1]. It is estimated that one in six deaths globally is due to cancer, which equates to 10 million cancer deaths per year [2, 3]. Despite the incidence of cancer being higher in high-income countries (HICs), it is predicted that by 2030, 75% of global cancer deaths will occur in LMICs [4]. The most common cancers worldwide include breast, lung, bowel and prostate cancers (Fig. 16.1).

16.2 Why Are the Number of New Cancer Cases Increasing Globally?

Cancer incidence and mortality are rapidly increasing worldwide [5]. There are many complex reasons for this, some include:

- An ageing population—increasing population size, increasing life expectancy and reduced family size are leading to an older population demographic in many high-income countries
- Increasing global population size
- Previous focus on other major causes of death

U. Barclay · O. Curtis-Hughes · M. Evans · H. Raval (✉)
School of Medicine, Cardiff University, Cardiff, UK
e-mail: barclayu@cardiff.ac.uk; curtis-hughesog@cardiff.ac.uk;
evansmc1@cardiff.ac.uk; hannah.raval@doctors.org.uk

© The Author(s), under exclusive license to Springer Nature   151
Switzerland AG 2024
A. Fiander, G. Fry (eds.), *A Healthcare Students Introduction to Global Health*,
https://doi.org/10.1007/978-3-031-66563-9_16

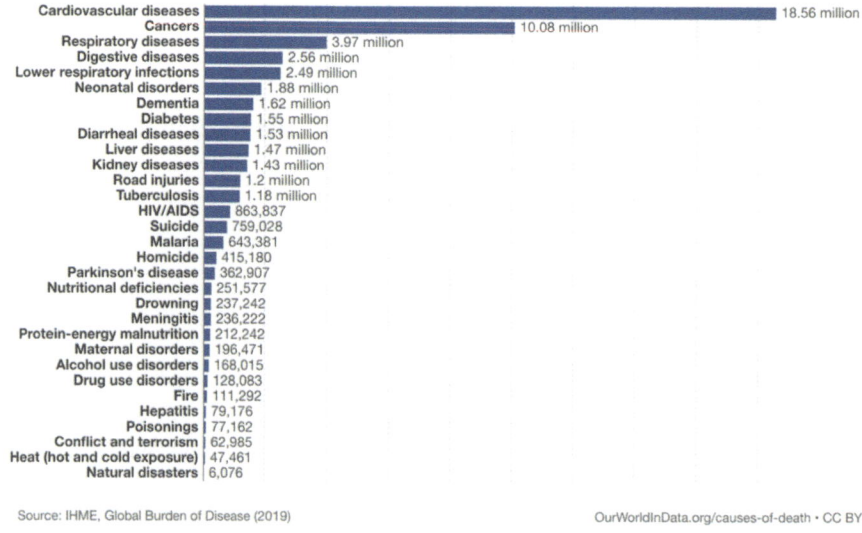

Causes of death, World, 2019

The estimated annual number of deaths from each cause. Estimates come with wide uncertainties, especially for countries with poor vital registration[1] .

Source: IHME, Global Burden of Disease (2019)   OurWorldInData.org/causes-of-death · CC BY

1. **Civil and Vital Registration System**: A Civil and Vital Registration System (CVRS) is an administrative system in a country that manages information on births, marriages, deaths and divorces. It generates and stores 'vital records' and legal documents such as birth certificates and death certificates. You can read more about how deaths are registered around the world in our article: How are causes of death registered around the world?

Fig. 16.1 Number of deaths by cause, World, 2019 [1]

- Increased exposure to lifestyle-associated cancer risk factors. For example, obesity, tobacco use, alcohol consumption and physical inactivity are associated with one-third of cancer-associated deaths
- Improved detection and surveillance in HICs lead to more cancer cases being identified.

16.3   What Does the Future Look Like?

In 2020, there were 18 million new cancer cases globally. Cancer Research UK has predicted that if recent trends continue, there will be 28 million new cases of cancer globally each year by 2040 [6]. Overall, 30–50% of cancer cases could have been prevented by:

- Avoiding or modifying key risk factors, e.g. smoking is the single biggest preventable cause of death worldwide.
- Implementing and maintaining prevention strategies, e.g. human papillomavirus and hepatitis B vaccinations.

Many cancers are curable if detected early and treated appropriately. Organisations such as the WHO are therefore collaborating with governments on strategies against cancer, particularly in LMICs.

The causes of death vary significantly across the globe. In high-income countries, 2 of the top 10 causes of death are due to cancer (lung and bowel cancer), whereas in low-income countries (LICs), individual cancers are not featured in the top 10 causes of death. Despite a general decline, people in LICs are still more likely to die of a communicable disease (i.e. infectious disease) than a non-communicable disease.

Although the incidence of cancer is higher in HIC, improved cancer services for early detection, diagnosis and treatment mean that the overall risk of mortality from cancer is lower in HIC. LMIC health systems may struggle to provide accessible, adequate and affordable cancer care [5]. In 2017, less than 30% of LMICs reported that cancer treatments were readily available compared to 90% in HICs [6]. This contributes to the prediction that by 2030, 75% of global cancer deaths occur in LMICs [4].

16.4   What Are the Most Common Types of Cancer?

Globally, the most common types of cancer are:

- Lung cancer
- Breast cancer
- Colorectal cancer
- Prostate cancer
- Stomach cancer

In 2020, there were 10 million cancer-related deaths worldwide [6]. Lung, bowel, liver, stomach and prostate cancers cause the most cancer-related deaths in men worldwide, with breast, lung, bowel and cervical cancer causing the greatest number of deaths in women (Fig. 16.2).

The incidence of cancer types varies significantly across the globe in accordance with infectious diseases. In HICs, cancers like breast, lung and prostate are more common; however, in LMICs, cancers which are related to chronic infections are more prevalent. For example, cervical cancer related to the human papillomavirus (HPV) and Hepatitis B/C is a major cause of liver cancer. It is thought that viruses cause up to 30% of cancer cases in LMICs [2]. The attributable fraction of cancer related to infection is significantly higher in LMICs than HICs such as the UK, as shown in Fig. 16.3 [8].

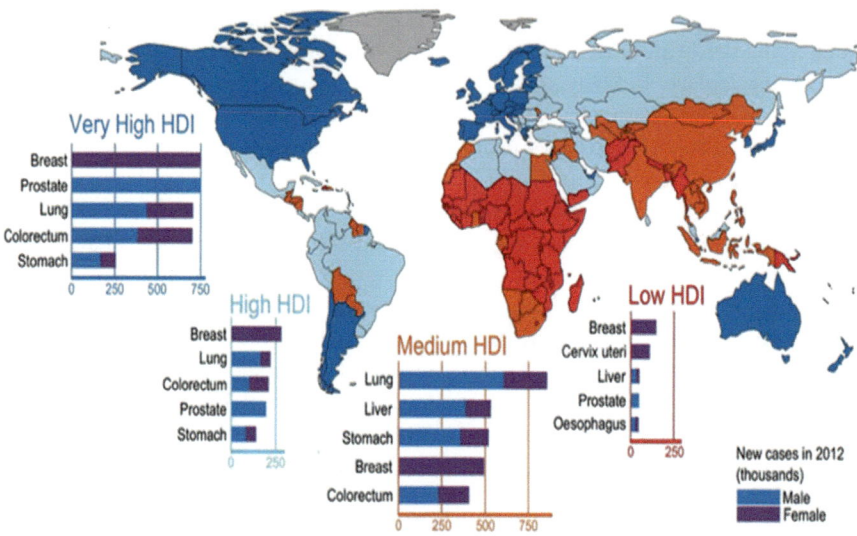

Fig. 16.2 The five most common cancers in 2012 according to levels of the Human Development Index (HDI) across the 184 countries included in GLOBOCAN [7]

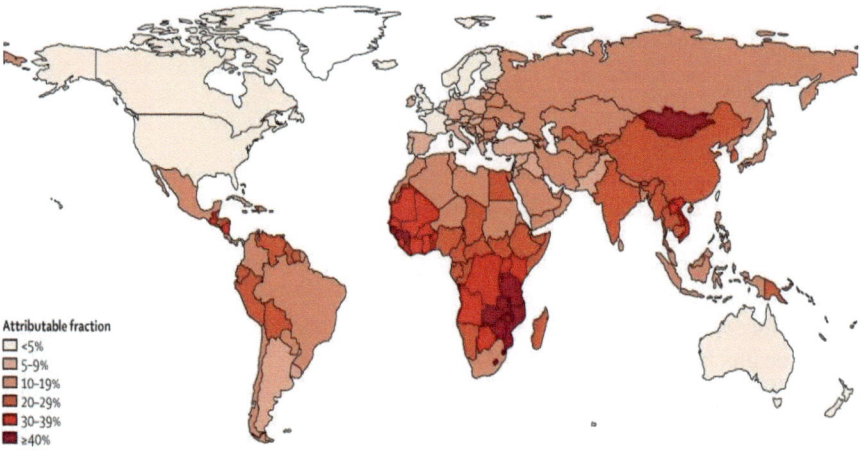

Fig. 16.3 Attributable fraction of cancer related to infection, 2012 [8]

16.5 Cervical Cancer

Cervical cancer is the fourth most common cancer in women. In 2020, the WHO recorded over 300,000 female cervical cancer deaths worldwide, with 90% of these deaths being in LMICs [9]. Cervical cancer has the largest inter-country range variation [10], which is mostly attributed to its rates of the HPV virus. In addition to this, women living with HIV are 6 times more likely to develop cervical cancer.

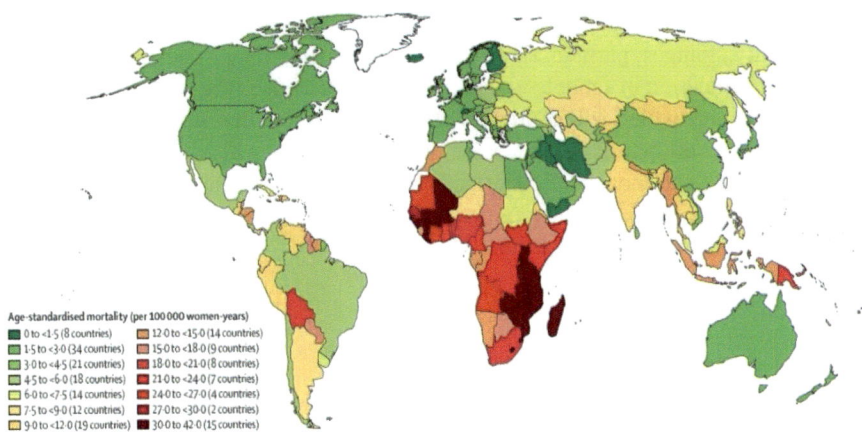

Fig. 16.4 Geographical distribution of world age-standardised mortality rate of cervical cancer by country, estimated for 2018 [10]

HPV is a sexually transmitted infection (STI) that has multiple strains, some cancer-causing and others not. Type 16 and 18 are 'high-risk strains' and cause around 70% of cervical cancers and pre-cancerous lesions.

The HPV vaccine provides protection against several strains and is routinely offered to 12–13-year-old girls and boys in countries such as the UK. Unfortunately, many LMICs do not offer an HPV vaccination programme, leaving their population particularly at risk of developing cervical cancers and genital warts. Furthermore, many LMICs do not offer a regular cervical screening programme, such as we do in the UK, resulting in women presenting with much more advanced cervical disease (Fig. 16.4).

16.6 Preventing Cancer in LMICs

16.6.1 Education

One-third of cancer deaths can be linked to lifestyle factors, including poor diet, lack of physical activity, tobacco use and alcohol consumption. Through the demographic transition and urbanisation, we are seeing many LMIC countries change their lifestyles to a more western, sedentary lifestyle. Through cultural globalisation, western 'fast food' is considered a more modern diet and a symbol of status. The switch from a more traditional diet to a processed diet is leading to an increasing global trend in obesity. Therefore, education about a healthy lifestyle is a vital method in cancer prevention, which can be easily implemented and at a low cost. However, when it comes to cancer prevention through a healthy diet, restricted food availability and choice within their local area may impede individuals' abilities to make dietary changes, particularly in LMICs where food may be scarce.

Starting education in schools will encourage the practice of good lifestyle habits from a young age which will continue into adulthood. Healthy lifestyle choices can be promoted on billboards in rural areas or on packaging, which is particularly relevant to alcohol and tobacco. Education is needed regarding the risks of household air pollution from cooking on open fires in poorly ventilated areas, which is a contributing factor towards lung cancers.

16.6.2   Screening

Effective screening programmes can identify early signs of common cancers and result in prompt intervention, improving cancer outcomes. Screening programmes are targeted at specific 'at-risk groups' within the population. There can be significant barriers to patient access and uptake of these screening programmes. For example, travelling long distances to healthcare services or a lack of understanding of the benefits of screening. In addition, screening programmes are redundant and a waste of resources, if they are not accompanied by adequate diagnostic and treatment services.

16.6.3   Vaccination Programmes

The Hepatitis B vaccine has been rolled out across 190 countries, with a global coverage of 45%, however on 18% in parts of Africa. The HPV vaccine is part of the national immunisation service by 130 WHO member states; however, the global coverage is still only at 21% [11].

Vaccination programmes can be costly and logistically challenging, as seen with the COVID-19 vaccine roll out. Vaccine equity is a major issue, ensuring vaccines are equally distributed based on need and not economic status. In many LMICs, there are difficulties delivering vaccines in temperature-controlled environments, known as 'cold chains'. Therefore, people living in remote areas are doubly disadvantaged when it comes to vaccine equity.

16.7   What Are the Cost Implications for Treating Cancer?

According to the American Institute of Cancer Research, 'cancer costs the world more money than any other disease—about $895 billion a year'. Alongside drugs, that includes the costs of diagnosis, radiotherapy, imaging, pathology, surgery and end-of-life care.

Healthcare systems in many LMICs are not financially equipped to manage the increasing rate of cancer cases. Whilst an estimated 60% of cancer cases occur in LMICs, only 5% of global spending on cancer is directed at these countries. Commonly, the patient has to cover the majority of the cost of their own cancer care (out-of-pocket expenditure) with little governmental contribution. This may be related to limited government budgets, where less money is prioritised towards healthcare.

Furthermore, lack of screening programmes and education regarding cancer symptoms results in patients presenting with more advanced disease. The cost of treatment is significantly higher for metastatic disease than if it is caught in the early stages. This is compounded by the lack of access to healthcare in many areas, resulting in delays with diagnosis and accessing treatment.

> **Case Example: Cost-Effectiveness of Screening and Treatment for Cervical Cancer in Tanzania [12]**
> Eighty-five per cent of cervical cancer cases occur in LMICs. In this study by Neslon et al. [12], the cost of treatment for cervical cancer was compared for women who had been diagnosed through screening and those who had not. Screening aims to increase early diagnoses, allowing for better treatment outcomes. However, screening services require significant resources and expense. This study concluded that despite these additional costs, it was overall more cost effective to implement a screening service than not, therefore highlighting the importance of expanding cervical cancer screening services to other LMIC settings.

16.7.1 Palliative Care

Palliative care plays a significant role in the management of cancers, focusing on symptom relief rather than cure. However, access to palliative care is lacking in many LMICs, where the infrastructure, funding or knowledge may not be available. Furthermore, the high burden of disease and lack of healthcare professionals often result in palliative care not being seen as a priority. In particular, access to adequate pain management is a big problem, where opioids are often stigmatised and may not be accepted culturally. Palliative care is one of the greatest disparities in global healthcare [12].

References

1. The top 10 causes of death [Internet]. [cited 2023 Sep 26]. Available from: https://www.who.int/news-room/fact-sheets/detail/the-top-10-causes-of-death
2. Cancer [Internet]. [cited 2023 Oct 3]. Available from: https://www.who.int/news-room/fact-sheets/detail/cancer

3. Cancer (IARC) TIA for R on. Global Cancer Observatory [Internet]. [cited 2023 Oct 3]. Available from: https://gco.iarc.fr/
4. Lancet T. GLOBOCAN 2018: counting the toll of cancer. Lancet. 2018;392(10152):985.
5. Bray F, Ferlay J, Soerjomataram I, Siegel RL, Torre LA, Jemal A. Global cancer statistics 2018: GLOBOCAN estimates of incidence and mortality worldwide for 36 cancers in 185 countries. CA Cancer J Clin. 2018;68(6):394–424.
6. Cancer Research UK [Internet]. 2015 [cited 2023 Sep 27]. Worldwide cancer statistics. Available from: https://www.cancerresearchuk.org/health-professional/cancer-statistics/worldwide-cancer
7. Stewart BW, Bray F, Forman D, Ohgaki H, Straif K, Ullrich A, et al. Cancer prevention as part of precision medicine: 'plenty to be done'. Carcinogenesis. 2016;37(1):2–9.
8. Global burden of cancers attributable to infections in 2012: a synthetic analysis—The Lancet Global Health [Internet]. [cited 2023 Sep 28]. Available from: https://www.thelancet.com/journals/langlo/article/PIIS2214-109X(16)30143-7/fulltext
9. Cervical cancer [Internet]. [cited 2023 Sep 28]. Available from: https://www.who.int/news-room/fact-sheets/detail/cervical-cancer
10. Arbyn M, Weiderpass E, Bruni L, de Sanjosé S, Saraiya M, Ferlay J, et al. Estimates of incidence and mortality of cervical cancer in 2018: a worldwide analysis. Lancet Glob Health. 2020 Feb;8(2):e191–203.
11. Immunization coverage [Internet]. [cited 2023 Oct 1]. Available from: https://www.who.int/news-room/fact-sheets/detail/immunization-coverage
12. Poudel A, Kc B, Shrestha S, Nissen L. Access to palliative care: discrepancy among low-income and high-income countries. J Glob Health. 9(2):020309.

Chapter 17
Palliative Care in Low Resource Countries

Emily Finn and Evan Maher

17.1 The Principles of Palliative Care

Palliative care seeks to improve the quality of life of both patients and families suffering the effects of life-threatening and complex illness [1]. It is intended to relieve suffering and focuses on a holistic approach to care.

Palliative care does not simply focus on the physical but also encompasses psychological, social and spiritual support (Fig. 17.1). Palliative care is suitable at any time point over the course of an illness and can be provided in parallel to curative treatment or, in other circumstances, it can be the primary focus of care [2].

Palliative care incorporates the whole spectrum of care. A holistic approach, incorporating these wider aspects of care, is good medical practice, and in palliative care, it is essential [3].

Palliative care is distinct from end-of-life care. However, for patients suffering from terminal illness, as the end of life approaches, the importance of palliative care becomes increasingly significant.

Forty million people globally require palliative care each year, and 78% of these people live in low- and middle-income countries. This figure rises to 96% when considering children who require palliative care. Only 14% of those who need palliative care receive it, and most palliative care is provided in high-income countries [5]. In only 40% of countries worldwide do palliative care services reach half the population who require them.

E. Finn (✉) · E. Maher
School of Medicine, Cardiff University, Cardiff, UK
e-mail: finne1@cardiff.ac.uk; mahere2@cardiff.ac.uk

A. Fiander, G. Fry (eds.), *A Healthcare Students Introduction to Global Health*,
https://doi.org/10.1007/978-3-031-66563-9_17

Fig. 17.1 The 4
dimensions of palliative
care [4]

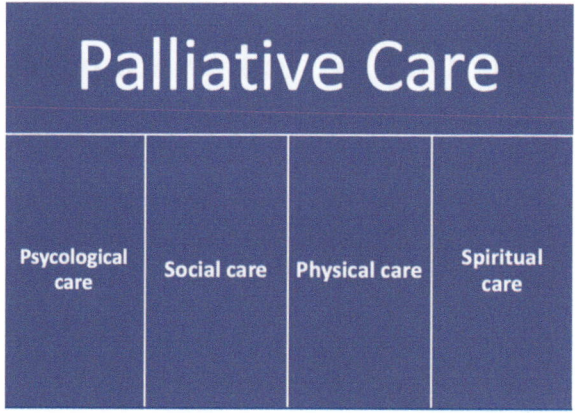

17.2   The Clinical Principles of Palliative Care

Appropriate palliative care should be specific to the illness stage of the individual, and thus, palliative care is extremely fluid and changes constantly. When treating an individual, care must be taken to ensure a humanistic approach, and a team approach is vital. Each team member may be able to observe various aspects of the patient's personality and suffering, and so can provide different insight into what is in their best interest.

Ensuring appropriate treatment is vital in palliative care, as mistakes or inappropriate treatment options can cause unnecessary suffering to an individual and their families. For example, the prescription of active therapy to treat the underlying disease. In this case, limitations to this therapy should be acknowledged, and the patient's condition should be monitored carefully to ensure the wishes of the patient are being adhered to.

Another key aspect of palliative care is to recognise that prolonging life is not necessarily the focus of care. Efforts instead must be directed towards relief of suffering and enhancing the quality of life of the patient. A focus on length of life may cause unnecessary discomfort to the individual and require invasive or traumatic treatment options which have little impact on the quality of life of the patient.

When considering the palliative care of an individual, thought must be given to their individual and cultural practices. The individual wishes of the patient, whether for personal, cultural or religious reasons, must be respected and prioritised even if they conflict with what is deemed by the palliative care team to be the best course of treatment. This personal aspect of palliative care treatment is something that is extremely important and must always be considered. This principle applies equally to the choice of the site of treatment for the patient, as many patients prefer home treatment wherever possible.

17.3   Palliative Care in the Context of Low Resource Countries

LRCs are facing a sharp rise in the prevalence of non-communicable diseases, for example cancer and cardiovascular disease [6]. Therefore, the need for effective palliative care services is becoming increasingly important. However, current palliative care provisions are inadequate, and this contributes to a complex set of issues ranging from undue suffering to economic difficulties.

Currently, there is a lack of integration of palliative care into national health systems in LRCs [7]. The lack of progress can be attributed to a misunderstanding of the meaning of palliative care, a lack of economic funding, and cultural and religious beliefs surrounding death. These issues have slowed progress significantly in LRCs, and work is currently being undertaken by numerous groups to combat this.

In low resource settings, a lack of palliative care places a heavy burden on individuals, families and communities.

Individuals may face intense and prolonged suffering on account of lack of availability of analgesics. Oral opioid use is infrequent as there are concerns that increasing availability may worsen the problem of substance abuse.

The impact on families too can prove extensive. When a patient is no longer able to work due to illness, a lack of wages can threaten the livelihood of families already facing poverty (Fig. 17.2). Other members of the family may also be unable to work as they are caring for the patient. To fund healthcare or medication, families may resort to selling their homes, assets, for example livestock, or withdrawing children from school. This lack of education for children poses a barrier to social mobility and prevents children having the means to escape poverty, as well as negatively

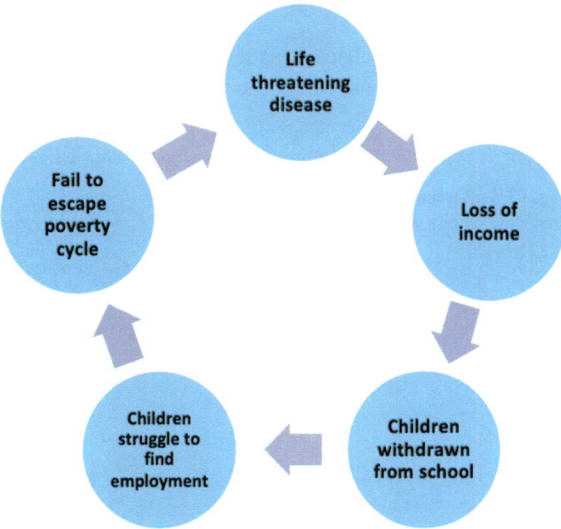

Fig. 17.2 Flow chart demonstrating the poverty cycle that results from a lack of palliative care provision [5]

impacting the local economy. Thus, a lack of palliative care in LRCs perpetrates a cycle of poverty [5].

17.4 Cost Effectiveness

Palliative care can take place in several settings, including in a patient's own home. This is less expensive when compared to hospital-based care. Community and home care is often preferred by patients and improves their quality of life. Where the same level of medical care can be provided in a setting outside of the hospital, this is preferable [8].

This is also beneficial as it reduces the pressure on health services, many of which are already overburdened and underfunded.

Palliative care also reduces the burden on caregivers. This means that relatives can still work and so reduces the financial impact of illness on families, helping families emancipate themselves from the cycle of poverty.

17.5 Barriers to Palliative Care in LRCs (Fig. 17.3)

• Shortage of trained staff to provide palliative care

The average vacancy rate for specialist palliative care nurses in the NHS 2010 was 8.7%, compared to just 0.6% for nurses in general. Thus, a clear shortage of trained staff in the NHS translates into an even greater shortage of trained staff in LRCs [9].

• Lack of availability of opioids or restrictions surrounding their use

Developing countries constitute 80% of the world's population, and yet, these countries only receive 6% of the world's morphine [9].

Fig. 17.3 Barriers to provision of palliative care in LRCs [5]

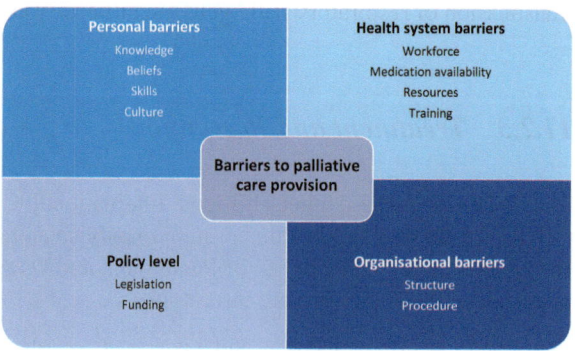

- Cultural attitudes of both healthcare staff and patients

For example, there is a common belief that the use of opioids for palliative care purposes will automatically lead to addiction, and so their use is often avoided [9].

- Lack of funding for palliative care resources

A systematic review found that 5 of the 14 papers concluded that a lack of funding was the greatest barrier to providing adequate palliative care in LRCs [9].

- Language barriers

Globally, there are limited guidelines for establishing palliative care systems in LRCs. Where these guidelines do exist, they are routinely only available in five translated languages: Bengali, French, Mandarin, Portuguese and Spanish. Thus, this limits the effectiveness of the guidelines in countries where these languages are not routinely spoken [7].

17.6 Tackling the Problem of Inadequate Palliative Care

17.6.1 Hospice Africa

Hospice Africa is a provider of palliative care and palliative care training in Africa. It was founded in 1992 and developed a model of culturally acceptable and affordable palliative care which could be adapted and applied all over Africa (Fig. 17.4).

The clinical headquarters are in Uganda, and here, they treat patients, manufacture morphine and host education programmes.

The education department provides undergraduate training programmes for nurses, doctors and other healthcare providers. Students from all over Africa can take part in palliative care study programmes and subsequently take their new knowledge back to their own countries (Fig. 17.5).

This allows palliative care skills to be developed all over Africa [10].

17.6.2 Asia Pacific Hospice Palliative Care Network

It is a charitable organisation dedicated to hospice and palliative care in Asia and the Pacific.

The network was developed over a series of meetings between 1995 and 2001 hosted in Japan, where palliative care experts from across these regions came together to discuss the challenges they were facing whilst providing palliative care.

The network promotes training and education in palliative care, allowing countries across Asia and the Pacific to establish their own rigorous and sustainable palliative care system.

Fig. 17.4 Hospice Africa logo [10]

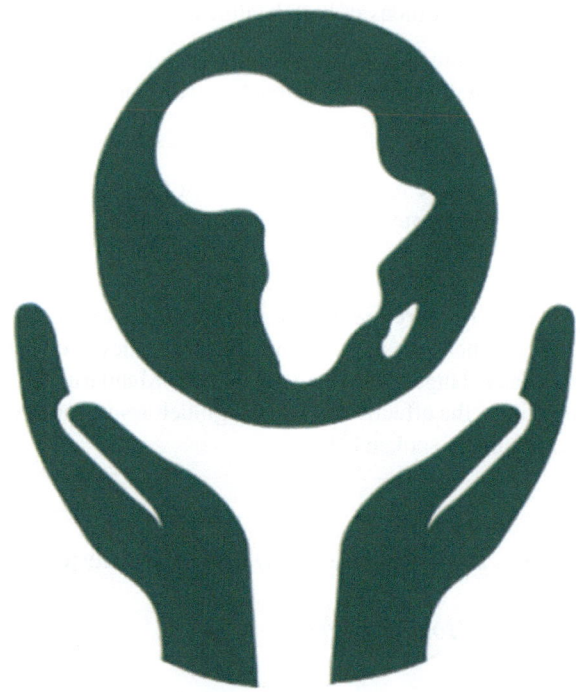

Fig. 17.5 Hospice Africa statistics [11]

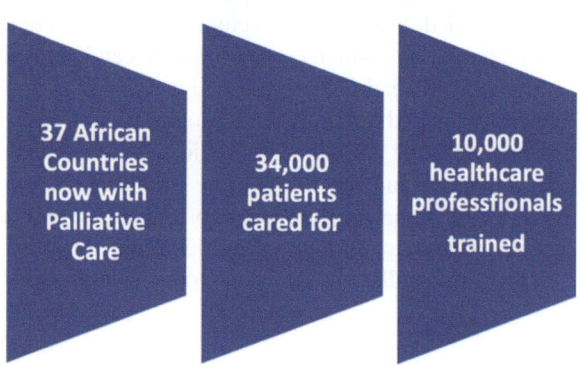

The network also works to promote research and collaboration between countries in these regions to ensure the continuing improvement of palliative care services.

References

1. World Health Organisation. Palliative Care [Internet]. 2020 [cited 2020 Nov 10]. Available from: https://www.who.int/news-room/fact-sheets/detail/palliative-care

2. Rome RB et al. The role of palliative care at the end of life. Ochsner J [Internet] 2011;11(4):348–52. Available from: https://www.ncbi.nlm.nih.gov/pmc/articles/ PMC3241069/
3. International Association for Hospice and Palliative Care. Principles of palliative care [Internet]. 2020 [cited 2020 Nov 10]. Available from: https://hospicecare.com/what-we-do/ publications/getting-started/principles-of-palliative-care/
4. University of Edinburgh. All dimensions of need [Internet]. 2016 [cited 2020 Nov 10]. Available from: https://www.ed.ac.uk/usher/primary-palliative-care/themes/all-dimensions-of-need
5. Anderson RE, Grant L. What is the value of palliative care provision in low-resource settings? BMJ Global Health [Internet] 2017;2(1). Available from: https://gh.bmj.com/ content/2/1/e000139
6. Basu A, Mittag-Leffler BN, Miller K. Palliative care in low- and medium-resource countries [internet]. Cancer J. 2013;19(5):410–3. Available from: https://pubmed.ncbi.nlm.nih. gov/24051614/
7. Cruz-Oliver DM, Little MO, Woo J, Morley JE. End-of-life care in low- and middle-income countries [Internet]. Bull World Health Organ. 2017;95(11):731. Available from: https://www. ncbi.nlm.nih.gov/pmc/articles/PMC5677606/
8. Public Health England. Understanding the health economics of palliative and end of life care. London: Public Health England; 2017. Available from: https://assets.publishing.service.gov. uk/government/uploads/system/uploads/attachment_data/file/612377/health-economics- palliative-end-of-life-care.pdf
9. Abu-Odah H, Molassiotis A, Liu J. Challenges on the provision of palliative care for patients with cancer in low- and middle-income countries: a systematic review of reviews. BMC Palliat Care 2020 [cited 2020 Nov 10]; 19:55. Available from: https://bmcpalliatcare.biomedcentral. com/articles/10.1186/s12904-020-00558-5
10. Hospice Africa. Palliative Care for Africa [Internet]. 2020 [cited 2020 Nov 10]. Available from: https://www.hospice-africa.org/
11. Asia Pacific Hospice Palliative Care Network. Who We Are [Internet]. 2020 [cited 2020 Nov 11]. Available from: https://aphn.org/who-we-are/#:~:text=The%20Asia%20Pacific%20 Hospice%20Palliative,suffering%20from%20life%2Dthreatening%20illness

Chapter 18
Disability in Low Resource Countries

Nathan White and Madeleine Mills

18.1 Introduction

The International Classification of Functioning, Disability and Health (ICF) defines disability as an umbrella term for impairment in body function or structure, activity limitation and participation restriction [1]. It is the interaction between the individual with the health condition, e.g. Down's syndrome or depression, and personal and environmental factors, e.g. negative attitudes and limited social support.

Disability may be a physical or mental condition, and it is heavily affected by social and physical barriers which may be more common or severe in low resource countries (LRCs).

The rates of disability are increasing due to an ageing population and increased prevalence of chronic disease.

18.2 Did You Know

Sixteen per cent of people have some form of a disability across the globe [2].

Visual Impairment affects 2.2 billion people globally, and it is neglected in at least 1 billion sufferers with LRC residents being 4 times more likely to be affected [3].

N. White · M. Mills (✉)
Cardiff University, Cardiff, UK
e-mail: whitenp@cardiff.ac.uk; millsm2@cardiff.ac.uk

© The Author(s), under exclusive license to Springer Nature Switzerland AG 2024
A. Fiander, G. Fry (eds.), *A Healthcare Students Introduction to Global Health*, https://doi.org/10.1007/978-3-031-66563-9_18

⚕️ One in 20 of the global population requires treatment for hearing loss with 4 out of 5 people living with disabling hearing loss living in low and middle resource countries [4].

👩 Women, young children and the elderly are more likely to experience disability [5].

18.3   How Do We Measure Disability?

Disability-adjusted life years (DALYs) are a standard used to quantify disease burden across conditions and allow us to compare different diseases as well as evaluate and monitor treatment or prevention strategies.

DALYs are defined as 'the sum of years of potential life lost due to premature death and the years of productive life lost due to disability compared to a standardized life expectancy'. The WHO describes one DALY as the equivalent of 'one year of "healthy" life lost'. A DALY can be calculated using the following formula [6]:

$$DALY = YLD \left(\begin{array}{c} \text{"Years Lost due to Disability for incident cases} \\ \text{of the health condition"} \end{array} \right)$$
$$+ YLL \left(\text{"years of life lost due to premature mortality"} \right)$$

You can calculate DALYs for an individual or for an entire population.

YLL is calculated using the formula: $YLL = N * L$ (N = number of deaths and L = standard life expectancy at age of death).

YLD is calculated using the formula: $YLD = I * DW * L$ (I = number of incident cases, DW = disability weight, L = average duration of the case until remission or death (in years)).

The below calculations are simplified and do not include age weighting or discounting.

18.3.1   Calculation for an Individual

Let's look at an example for an individual: For example, a man dies of a lung disease at 45 when his life expectancy is 55.

Mortality is the Years of Life Lost compared to life expectancy.

$$55 - 45 = 10$$

Morbidity is also calculated. Let's say he spent 10 years with this condition with a disability weight of 0.4.

$$0.4 \times 10 = 4$$

This man's DALYs will therefore be $10 + 4 = 14$.

18.3.2 Calculation for a Population

Now let's look on a Population level:

In this example, 500 people die of a heart condition with an average age of 68 in a region where the life expectancy is usually 75.

Mortality assesses Years of Life Lost (YLL) = number of deaths multiplied by (life expectancy—age of death)

$$YLL = 500 \times (75 - 68) = 3500$$

Morbidity now considers the Years Lived with Disability.

In this example, our theoretical data finds the following: in a timeframe, 500 people are found to have the heart condition with a disability weighting of 0.3 and an average length of condition of 10 years.

$$YLD = \text{incidence} \times \text{Disability weighting} \times \text{mean length} \\ \text{of a condition until death or remission.}$$

$$YLD = 500 \times 0.3 \times 10 = 1500$$

DALYS in this population therefore equate to $3500 + 1500 = 5000$.

DALYs are used to represent a 'health gap', meaning the difference between the current state of a population's health and the ideal state in which every individual lives to the standard life expectancy and in good health. Effective treatments can reduce the impact of disability and prolong life, thus reducing DALYs and the burden of disease. The same can be said for prevention programmes such as screening and vaccination. Using DALYs, it is then possible to assess the efficacy of certain interventions and for organisations, such as the WHO, to target funding and support accordingly.

DALYs do have some flaws however, as they may not fully appreciate the nuances of how multiple conditions interact or the environmental impact on disease burden. Instead, they utilise a broad and generalised approach. A visual representation of how the concept of a DALY is made can be seen below in Fig. 18.1.

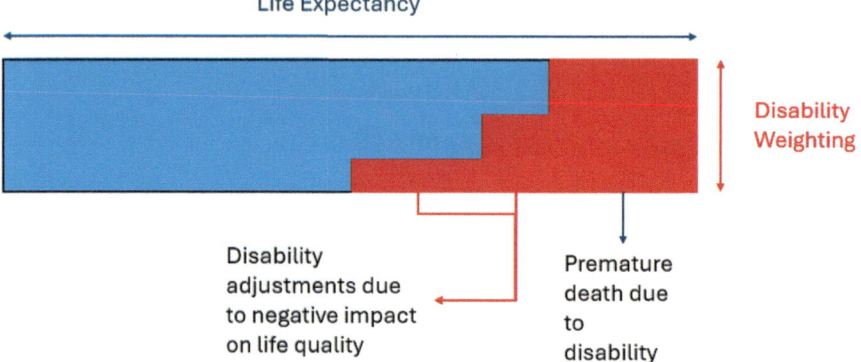

Fig. 18.1 A graphical representation of how morbidity as disability weighting and years of life lost as mortality combine to calculate DALYs

18.4 Different Types of Disability, Their Causes and Effects

There are multiple forms of disability, and the effect they have on patients is individualistic. An overview of the common reasons for and consequences of disability is summarised in Fig. 18.2. Effects should be contextualised to a patient's psychological, social and community factors.

Types of Disability
- Physical

  - Effects: Limb defects can make mobility and basic functions like washing and eating difficult.
  - Causes: Traumatic amputations can be caused by work accidents or armed conflict. Other causes include progressive neurological diseases.

- Sensory

  - Effects: Sensory disabilities can greatly impact a person's social interactions with communication barriers disrupting their education and relationships.
  - Causes: Blindness and deafness can be caused by congenital infections such as Rubella or acquired later in life due to other pathology.

- Mental Health

  - Effects: Mental health is often stigmatised in many countries and can be considered as demonic possession. It can have a severe impact on jobs and relationships.
  - Causes: Mental health may be related to Adverse Childhood Events (ACEs) or regions of conflict.

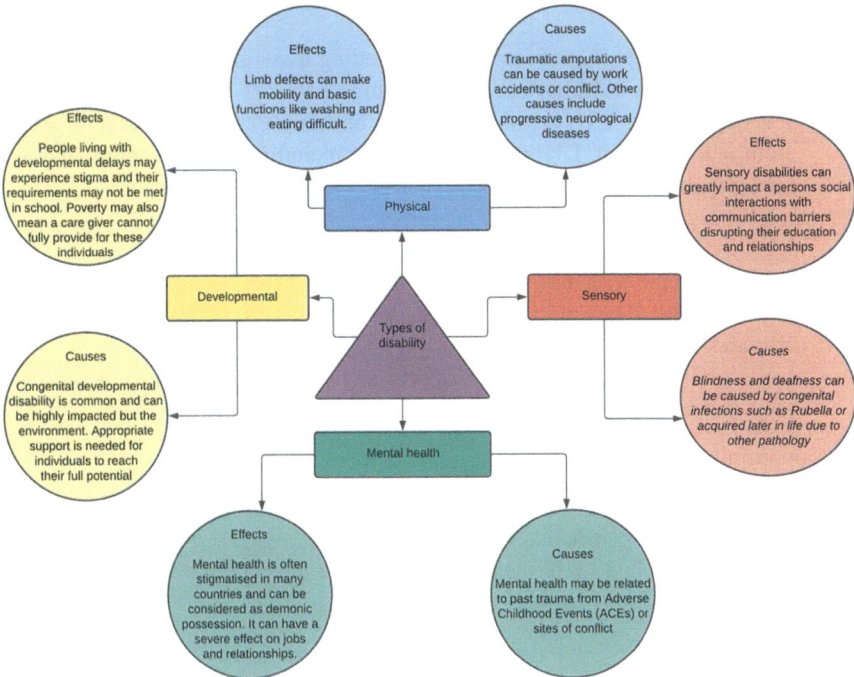

Fig. 18.2 A graphical overview of categories of disability summarized in four primary focuses

- Developmental
  - Effects: People living with developmental delays may experience stigma and their requirements may not be met in school. Poverty may also mean a care giver cannot fully provide for these individuals.
  - Causes: Congenital developmental disability is common and can be highly impacted by the environment. Appropriate support is needed for individuals to reach their full potential.

Barriers Affecting Disability in LRCs
- Poverty
  - Cost: People living with disability may not be able to afford suitable nutrition or medical care due to direct or associated costs such as transport. In LRCs, over half of people with a disability cannot afford healthcare compared to a third in those without disability.
  - Inadequate infrastructure: Medical support may be too far away or difficult to get to. Insufficient funding or resources mean people cannot get the help they need.

- Access
  - Healthcare: Only 5 to 15% of people needing assisting devices such as hearing, or mobility aids, have access to them in LRCs.
  - Physical Barriers: Travel or insufficient building design can prevent people from reaching care. Diagnostic equipment including mammograms may not have capability for specific needs such as wheelchair users.

- Social
  - Stigma: People with disability are at an increased risk of abuse and safeguarding concerns. They may be unable to access support due to community attitudes.
  - Isolation: Due to lack of social support, individuals may not be able to reach their full potential in work or education.

- Opportunity
  - Jobs: Disabled people may only have access to informal employment due to lack of training or education.
  - Education: Only 10% of disabled students are in school, and only one in five of these finishes primary school.

18.5 What Is the Burden of Disability for Global Health?

Chronic disease is becoming more common, and most of the disease burden has shifted from communicable diseases (e.g. malaria) to non-communicable diseases (e.g. cardiovascular disease). Due to advances in healthcare, we have a globally ageing population which leads to more 'Years Lived with Disability' (YLDs). As stated in the Lancet [7], healthcare infrastructures must be invested in and adapted to address the increasingly ageing population and complexity of chronic conditions. Economies should also anticipate more suffering from disabilities, which may lead to a loss in capital. Low resource countries may struggle to supply the healthcare required to people with disabilities.

18.6 Why Do the Poor Suffer More Disability?

Poverty and disability are inherently linked in a vicious cycle. Both factors feed into and worsen each other, making it extremely difficult for people with disabilities in poverty to thrive. Let's take a look at how and what can be done to help.

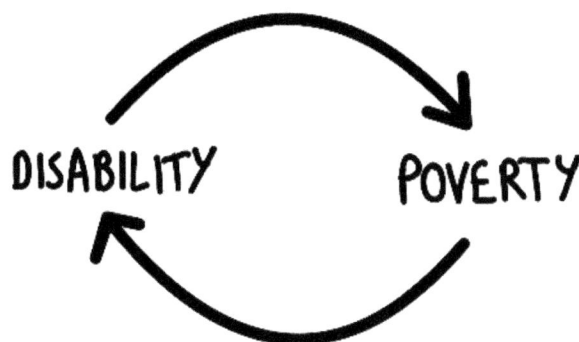

People in poverty are at an increased risk of disability due to:

- *Reduced access to suitable nutrition*: Poor maternal nutrition is described as a BMI <18.5. It can stunt foetal development in utero. Fifteen per cent of babies globally have a low birth weight. A subsequent low birth weight in this critical developmental phase is associated with worse health outcomes later in life [8]. A maternal diet lacking in folate (Vitamin B9) can also put the developing foetus at increased risk of neural tube defects such as spina bifida [9].
- *Increased risk of accidents and work-related injury*: LRCs such as Tanzania may rely on certain potentially dangerous job industries. These can include agriculture, mining and manufacturing. Poor training and less stringent health and safety regulations result in accidents at work being more common. Road traffic collisions are also frequent in LRCs with 90% of DALYS from road traffic accidents occurring in LRCs [10]. Poor countries may also be at an increased risk of internal conflict from civil war or terror-related groups.
- *Lack of clean water and sanitation*: Poor water and sanitation can lead to the development of conditions such as parasitic disease, schistosomiasis and diarrhoeal disease. Around the world 780 million don't have access to clean drinking water, and young children in LRCs have an average of three diarrhoeal episodes a year, placing them at risk of dehydration [11].
- *Poor healthcare*: As mentioned previously, there are many barriers to accessing healthcare such as distance, stigma and cost. One study in rural South Africa, a middle-income country, shows people with disability are almost twice as likely to report they did not get the healthcare they needed. This was mainly due to lack of safe transport, inadequate drugs or equipment, and the general absence of the services that they required [12].

18.7   How Does Disability Cause or Trap People in Poverty?

- *Difficulty accessing education*: Disability can make it more difficult for a child or adult to access a decent education. In some LRCs, teachers do not have inclusivity and equality training, meaning many students with disabilities do not receive the support they need to reach their full potential. Some educators also have limited experiences with disability and may not believe the individual is capable or wanting to learn. Together, this has led to millions of children being denied the basic human right of education [13].
- *Discrimination in the workplace*: In some countries, up to 80% of disabled people who are capable of work are unemployed [14]. Due to stigma and social isolation, a disabled individual may not be given the same opportunities of employment or promotion within the workplace. These factors have led to a high proportion of disabled people working in the informal sector.
- *LRC focused barriers to inclusion of disabled people*: Further factors are summarised below in the infographic seen in Fig. 18.3. As detailed above, the intricate link between poverty and disability can create a vicious cycle. These barriers can be multifactorial and interlink with one another.

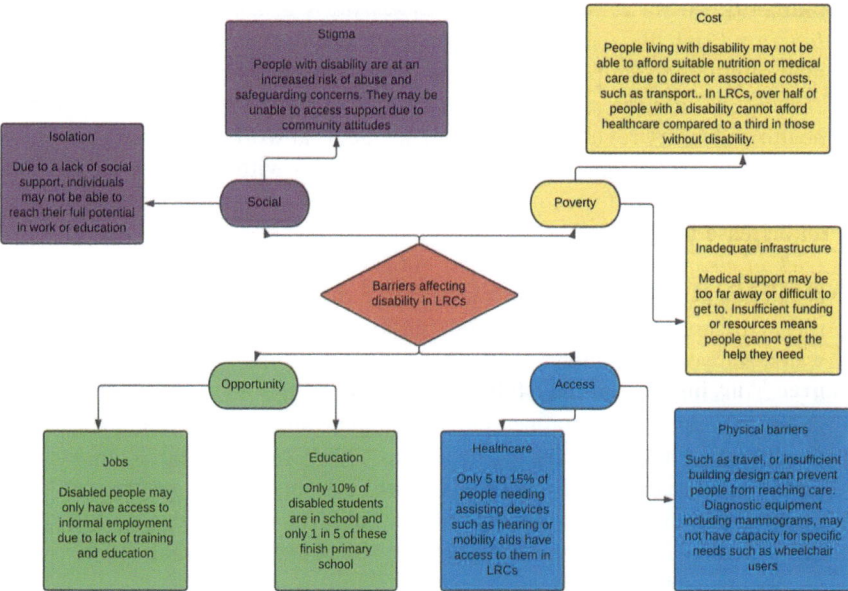

Fig. 18.3 A diagram suggesting ways people living with disability may face inequality or be discriminated against (Created in Lucidchart). Facts and figures in diagram from lecture presented by Sian Tensi [15]

18.8 How Can Disability in LRCs Be Addressed?

- On a community level, it is vital to *improve awareness and education* about disability. This will help to reduce stigma, improve diagnosis and management.
- There should be better *provision of disability benefits and financial support* for those with disability as research shows that they are more likely to live in poverty.
- Governments should *adapt healthcare services* to cater to people with disabilities. For example, improving access, physical layout of facilities and the use of Braille. Improving the general health of the population and disease eradication (e.g. leprosy) would further reduce the prevalence of disability.
- If countries *adopt the International Classification of Functioning, Disability and Health (ICF)*, they can keep records of the physical, mental and social aspects of the patient's condition [16]. The health professional can then plan interventions to improve quality of life.
- Improve *national disability statistics* and fill research gaps.
- Address policies and legislation to comply with the *Convention on the Rights of Persons with Disabilities* (CRPD) [17]. This will establish better healthcare standards for people with disabilities.
- Widespread implementation of *Community-based rehabilitation* [18].

> The Convention on the Rights of Persons with Disability (CRPD) was established by the UN in 2006. It takes the movement from viewing persons with disabilities as 'objects' of charity, medical treatment and social protection towards viewing persons with disabilities as 'subjects' with rights, who are capable of making decisions based on informed consent as well as being active members of society.

18.9 What Is Community-Based Rehabilitation (CBR)?

CBR is a strategy that focuses on the capacity of communities themselves to help the rehabilitation, equalisation and social inclusion of people with disabilities [18]. It is implemented through the combined efforts of people with disabilities, their families, communities and the appropriate health, education and social services.

One of the benefits of CBR is that it can take place in rural areas with limited infrastructure. It is independent of government control and makes the most of community involvement to address local needs and make use of local resources. For example, mothers of children with cerebral palsy can be taught simple physiotherapy techniques in situations where there may not be professionally qualified healthcare professionals.

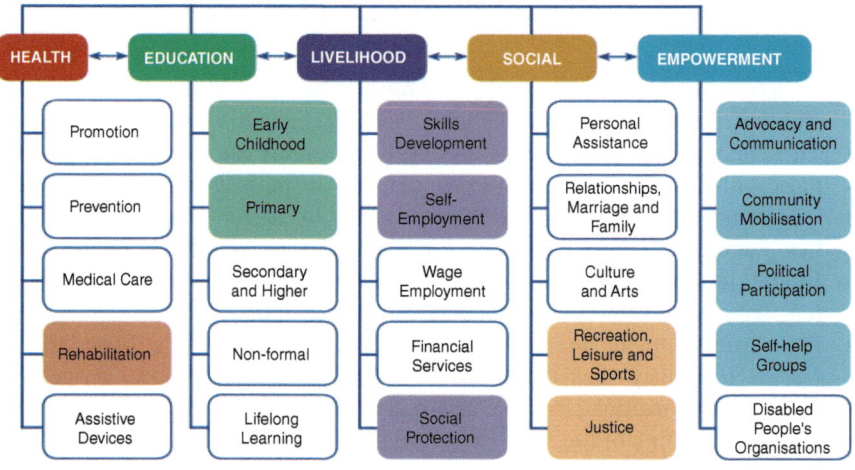

Fig. 18.4 A diagram reflecting the work of the Afrika Tikkun Empowerment Programme [19]

18.9.1 Case Study

One example of the CBR programme is the Afrika Tikkun Empowerment Programme [19]. It has three sites located across the townships in Gauteng, South Africa. Their main beneficiaries are orphans and vulnerable children with disabilities, but it also aims to support parents and caregivers.

The matrix in Fig. 18.4 shows the work of the Afrika Tikkun Empowerment programme. It allows us to think holistically about rehabilitation and assess progress made in each of the five components (health, education, livelihood, social and empowerment).

In this project, particular progress has been made in the 'Empowerment' component. This has consisted of educating children with disabilities on their rights, building self-help groups for caregivers and raising awareness of the abuse of children with disabilities.

18.10   What Is Being Done and How Can I Help?

Target 8.5 of the United Nations Sustainable Development Goals (SDGs) aims to achieve decent equal employment for all regardless of gender, age and disability by 2030, [20].

Never underestimate the power of your voice. You are needed as an advocate for disabled people across the globe. Get involved and share information about global projects that work closely with local communities to deliver what is needed and make the greatest impact. Follow and get inspired by the work of organisations such as Amnesty international. Most importantly, do your bit to tackle discrimination at home and abroad.

References

1. World Health Organization (WHO). International Classification of functioning, Disability and Health (ICF) [Internet]. World Health Organization; 2002 [cited 2020 Nov 12]. Available from: https://www.who.int/classifications/icf/icfbeginnersguide.pdf
2. World Health Organization (WHO). Disability [Internet]. World Health Organization; 2023 [cited 2023 Aug 18]. Available from: https://www.who.int/news-room/fact-sheets/detail/disability-and-health
3. World Health Organization (WHO). Vision Impairment and blindness [Internet]. World Health Organization; 2023 [cited 2023 Aug 28]. Available from: https://www.who.int/news-room/fact-sheets/detail/blindness-and-visual-impairment
4. World Health Organization (WHO). Deafness and hearing loss [Internet]. World Health Organization; 2023 [cited 2023 Aug 28]. Available from: https://www.who.int/news-room/fact-sheets/detail/deafness-and-hearing-loss
5. World Health Organization (WHO). World report on disability [Internet]. World health Organization; 2011 [cited 2023 Aug 18]. Available from: https://apps.who.int/iris/rest/bitstreams/53067/retrieve
6. Grosse SD, Lollar DJ, Campbell VA, Chamie M. Disability and disability-adjusted life years: not the same. Public Health Rep. 2009;124(2):197–202. https://doi.org/10.1177/003335490912400206.
7. Lancet T. The global burden of diseases: living with disability. Lancet. 2015;386(10009):2118. https://doi.org/10.1016/s0140-6736(15)01096-x.
8. Ahmed T, Hossain M, Sanin KI. Global burden of maternal and child undernutrition and micronutrient deficiencies. Ann Nutr Metab. 2012;61(Suppl. 1):8–17. https://doi.org/10.1159/000345165.
9. National Health Service (NHS). Vitamins, supplements and nutrition in pregnancy [Internet]. NHS; 2020 [cited 2023 Aug 18]. Available from: https://www.nhs.uk/pregnancy/keeping-well/vitamins-supplements-and-nutrition/
10. Nantulya VM. The neglected epidemic: road traffic injuries in developing countries. BMJ. 2002;324(7346):1139–41. https://doi.org/10.1136/bmj.324.7346.1139.
11. World Health Organization (WHO). Diarrhoeal disease [Internet]. World Health Organization; 2017 [cited 2012 Nov 12]. Available from: https://www.who.int/news-room/fact-sheets/detail/diarrhoeal-disease
12. Vergunst R, Swartz L, Hem K-G, Eide AH, Mannan H, MacLachlan M, et al. Access to health care for persons with disabilities in rural South Africa. BMC Health Serv Res. 2017;17(1) https://doi.org/10.1186/s12913-017-2674-5.
13. End The Cycle. Indepth: education, disability and poverty [internet]. YouTube; 2013 [cited 2020 Nov 12]. Available from: https://www.youtube.com/watch?v=ijRU4akqobM
14. International Labour Organization I. Facts on disability in the world of work [Internet]. 2007 [cited 2020 Nov 12]. Available from: https://www.ilo.org/asia/info/public/background/WCMS_098454/lang%2D%2Den/index.htm
15. Tensi S. Disability in LRCs [lecture to MBBCh medicine year 2 for Global Health SSC]. Cardiff University, 11 November 2020. Christoffel Blindenmission (CBM), sian. tesni@cbm.org

16. World Health Organization [WHO]. International Classification of Functioning, Disability and Health (ICF) 2020 [Accessed 30 Aug 2023]. Available from: https://www.who.int/standards/classifications/international-classification-of-functioning-disability-and-health
17. United Nations. Convention on the rights of persons with disabilities (CRPD). 2020 [accessed 30 Aug 2023]. Available from: https://www.un.org/development/desa/disabilities/convention-on-the-rights-of-persons-with-disabilities.html
18. AfriCAN. Community Based Rehabilitation (CBR). 2023 [Accessed 30 Aug 2023]. Available from: https://afri-can.org/
19. CBR Education and Training for Empowerment. Understanding community based rehabilitation in South Africa. South Africa: Creative Commons; 2015.
20. UNODC regional Office for Southeast Asia and the Pacific. Sustainable Development Goals 2015 [Accessed 30 Aug 2023]. Available from: https://www.unodc.org/roseap/en/sustainable-development-goals.html

Chapter 19
Conflict and Health

Isaac von Ruhland and Samuel Willis

Conflicts are acts of violence, between two or more parties, with the goal of enforcing compliance from the opposition. International Humanitarian Law (IHL), through the Geneva Conventions, defines an international armed conflict as that occurring between two or more opposing states, and a non-international armed conflict as that between non-governmental forces and either a governmental or another non-governmental force [1].

The nature of war has been both diverse and dynamic throughout human history. Whilst traditionally viewed from the perspective of the campaigns and battlefields of Europe between the sixteenth and nineteenth centuries and those of the American Civil War, the so-called 'old wars', the emergence of civil war, the War on Drugs with conflict with Cartels, the War on Terror and low-intensity conflict throughout the twentieth century, have led to the term 'new wars' [2], although these are not all unique to the modern era. Contemporary armed conflict is increasing in complexity due to the increasing magnitude of State and non-State participants, denial of involvement or disagreement as to whether a situation is defined as an armed conflict.

Prior to 1949, both the Geneva and Hague Conventions' conditions applied only to situations of declared war, whereby parties both acknowledged that a state of war existed between them. However, revisions of Article 2 at the 1949 Convention introduced the term 'armed conflict' when defining the settings in which Geneva Conventions apply, recognising the varied forms that armed conflicts take.

The impact of war extends far beyond the battlefield. It is a societal event with both direct and indirect effects on civilian populations due not only to combat-related injury and death, but through the disruption of infrastructure, breakdown in food and water supplies, outbreaks of disease epidemics and the formation of Refugee populations who experience their own unique health challenges.

I. von Ruhland · S. Willis (✉)
School of Medicine, Cardiff University, Cardiff, UK

A. Fiander, G. Fry (eds.), *A Healthcare Students Introduction to Global Health*, https://doi.org/10.1007/978-3-031-66563-9_19

19.1 Historical and Current Conflict

Debate exists surrounding the origins of armed conflict and warfare. Keith Otterbein, anthropologist and author on the topic of the origins of war, has posed two separate origins: the first, that of the violent encounters between hunter-gatherer peoples at the dawn of humankind, two million years ago; the second, that war evolved following the development of agriculture, a more complex human society with the emergence of city states, five to ten thousand years ago [3].

A change in the paradigm of armed conflict has occurred since the nineteenth century, with a shift from the national cross-border fronts and battlefields of the 'old wars' to a greater proximity to civilian life of modern conflict, bringing with it an increased toll on civilian populations and impact upon societal structure. Estimates of civilian casualties as a proportion of total lives lost have increased in this time frame, at 5% at the turn of the twentieth century, 15% throughout the First World War, 65% by the end of the Second World War and more than 90% in the wars of the 1990s [4]. These estimates, based on immediate mortality, do not account for non-combat-related deaths nor the post-war excess that occurs due to disrupted infrastructure [5, 6].

United Nations Secretary-General, António Guterres, at a meeting of the Peacebuilding Commission in March 2022 [7] reported that two billion people were living in conflict-affected areas, 84 million were forcibly displaced due to conflict, violence and human rights abuses, and that there would be an estimated 274 million requiring humanitarian assistance in that year. This was with the backdrop of the COVID-19 pandemic that had placed increasing restrictions on humanitarian access [8], and the Russian invasion of Ukraine, which triggered the largest refugee crisis since the Second World War.

Current, active armed conflicts are identified and monitored by The Rule of Law in Armed Conflicts (RULAC), an online portal through the Geneva Academy of International Humanitarian Law and Human Rights. Observation of situations where armed violence meets IHL definitions of armed conflict allows the theatres in which these laws apply to be identified. As of May 2023, there are more than 80 active armed conflicts being monitored, with over 50 States and 70 non-State organisations involved.

19.2 The Health Impact of Conflict

19.2.1 Conflict-Related Mortality

Morbidity and mortality during periods of armed conflict can be divided into:

1. Expected morbidity and mortality—unrelated to the conflict itself, but due to other factors such as disease, and is predicted from pre-conflict death rates.

2. Excess morbidity and mortality—both direct and indirect causes.

- Direct causes are combat-related injury and death and mostly affect adult males.
- Indirect causes are those due to subsequent epidemics, destruction of health-care infrastructure, disrupted food and water supply, and mostly affect the civilian population, in particular children.

The emergence and increasing incidence of infectious disease, malnutrition and deteriorating chronic healthcare provision all occur during wartime. Access to healthcare also becomes more challenging following the destruction of roads and displacement of people, and hospitals may become direct targets during military operations. Both acute and chronic healthcare challenges develop, with effects that continue far beyond the end to fighting.

19.2.2 Infectious Diseases

War and infectious disease are inseparable. Unsanitary conditions, close living proximity, poor nutrition and battle wounds have historically resulted in huge burdens on armed forces at war, with infectious disease having been termed 'the third army'. Approximately two-thirds of American Civil War soldiers' deaths were due to infectious disease [9], and a typhus epidemic halted Napoleon's 1812 Russian Campaign where half the French force was lost due to this infection [10].Whilst mortality of modern military personnel from infectious diseases is far lower than their historical counterparts, infectious disease is far from absent, with up to 50% of American soldiers developing acute diarrhoeal illness in Operations Desert Shield & Desert Storm of the Gulf War (1990–1991), and British forces experiencing many cases of pneumonia in that same conflict [11].

The causes of armed conflict are complex, involving factors such as conflicting political ideology, resource scarcity (be that actual or perceived), low GDP, natural disaster and intergroup mistrust. It has been proposed that infectious disease may also be contributory to civil war and intrastate conflict [12], in that it is not only an amplifier of the risk factors for conflict (low national wealth, depressed economic growth), but may act as a fissuring event between groups with differing localised immune defences to pathogens, with a resultant increase in mistrust between groups that is associated with increased intergroup conflict [13].

Infectious disease associated with armed conflict can be broadly categorised as:

1. Diseases associated with poor water, sanitation and hygiene (WASH).
2. Diseases associated with crowding.
3. Diseases associated with disrupted public health infrastructure.
4. Diseases of exploitation.

19.2.3   Disease Associated with Poor WASH

Short- and long-term disruption of WASH infrastructure occurs during conflict, resulting in an increased prevalence of gastrointestinal diseases. UNICEF's report Water Under Fire found that children in conflict zones are 20 times more likely to die due to diarrhoeal illness than violence in the conflict [14].

Cholera is associated with poor WASH, and outbreaks have been observed in several armed conflicts. A major epidemic developed in Yemen in 2016, one year following the outbreak of civil war in 2015 [15]. Increased rates of cholera outbreaks in Nigeria and the Democratic Republic of Congo of 3.6 and 2.6 times, respectively, have been observed during periods of armed conflict in these countries' histories between 1997 and 2020 [16, 17].

Whilst cholera is the most important disease associated with poor WASH, the incidence of other infections rises in areas of conflict. For example, intestinal helminth infections were present in 49% of paediatric patients hospitalised between 2012 and 2013 in the Gaza Strip during the Israeli occupation of 2012, exceeding that observed in previous years [18].

Case Example: Cholera Outbreaks of the Dadaab Refugee Complex, Kenya

The Dadaab Refugee Complex consists of three camps (Dagahaley, Hagadera and Ifo) in eastern Kenya, initially established in 1991 following civil war in Somalia, with a second large influx in 2011 following drought and famine in southern Somalia. As of July 2020, there was an officially registered population of 218,873; however, estimates have ranged from 300,000 to 400,000 occupants.

Several cholera outbreaks have occurred within the Dadaab complex and are often precipitated by heavy rains and flooding [19–22]. These rains and flooding result in:

1. A rapid influx of new refugees and asylum seekers from cholera endemic regions of Somalia.
2. Disruption to infrastructure maintaining safe, clean drinking water.

UNICEF Kenya has established an Integrated Cholera Response Plan to tackle these outbreaks consisting of increasing chlorination of water points, treating active cases with oral rehydration, or more intensive treatment at a cholera treatment centre, and community education projects surrounding good hygiene practices and safe water. Contact tracing and disease mapping is an important aspect of these responses.

Cholera outbreaks demonstrate the vulnerability of these refugee camps. The November 2011 outbreak was preceded by the arrival of an estimated 70,000 people in July and August following drought and famine in Somalia, straining the infrastructure of an already overcrowded environment. Between October 2022 and May 2023, nearly 3000 cholera cases had occurred in Dadaab following the breakdown of sanitation, where half of occupants do not have access to a functional latrine, and overcrowding. Over 1000 of these cases occurred in the Dagahaley camp, which hosts more that 140,000 individuals despite a capacity of 35,000.

19.2.4 Disease Associated with Crowding

Close living proximity, particularly in displaced peoples, and the breakdown of vaccination programmes set the stage for increased incidence of disease, particularly respiratory infections.

A massive diphtheria outbreak occurred in the overcrowded camp of Cox's Bazar, Bangladesh, among displaced Rohingya peoples, with over 7000 cases, the largest reported diphtheria outbreak in the refugee setting [23, 24]. Analysis of a diphtheria outbreak in Yemen 2017–2019 showed an 11-fold increase in cases in areas of active armed conflict [25].

Serial typhus epidemics, a disease spread by lice, fleas and chiggers, occurred throughout the squalid conditions of the ghettos and concentration camps of Nazi Germany. Deaths reached a peak of over 8500 at the Auschwitz concentration camp during the worst month of the 1942 Typhus epidemic [26] and over 3500 in the Warsaw Ghetto [27].

19.2.5 Disease Associated with Disrupted Public Health Infrastructure

Disrupted healthcare not only impacts upon the ability to deliver care to immediate health needs, but also the ability to conduct public health initiatives such as vaccination programmes, vector control and disease surveillance. Resources are also diverted from public health into military avenues, further exacerbating the stresses on the healthcare system.

Disrupted vector control led to the re-emergence of malaria following civil wars in Afghanistan (beginning in 1978) and in Tajikistan (1992–1997), a disease virtually eradicated prior to these events [28]. A total of 30,000 cases of malaria were recorded in 1997 in Tajikistan, rising to 100,000 a year in 2005, reflecting a persistent post-war effect.

Prevention and control of Ebola virus disease outbreaks in Eastern Democratic Republic of Congo through contact tracing and surveillance led to the end of a two and a half month Equateur Province outbreak, the ninth outbreak in the country.

However, 8 days after this declared end, a further outbreak occurred in the North Kivu Region following attacks on Ebola treatment centres and road blockades by armed groups [29]. The short period between outbreaks highlights the instability and challenges in disease control these regions face due to conflict. Tuberculosis morbidity and mortality also rise in conflict zones due to both delayed diagnosis and interrupted treatment, service closure, inability to access facilities and diverted resources, and have led to a series of epidemics in Ethiopia [30].

Polio outbreaks and re-emergence can be viewed as a marker of a failing health-care system. The marked success of the Global Polio Eradication Initiative has been threatened by armed conflict and the activity of armed groups. Areas free from polio for many decades observed an emergence of cases in 2013 in Syria, two years after the onset of civil war, spreading into neighbouring Iraq, attributed to a fall in polio immunisation rates [31].

19.2.6 Diseases of Exploitation

Sexual violence and exploitation are common during armed conflicts, with women and children often the victims of this. Despite the resultant poverty and infrastructure collapse that may accompany armed conflict, a direct relationship with HIV has not been demonstrated [32]. In populations with high pre-conflict HIV burdens, the added stressor of armed conflict exacerbates this burden. The decades-long conflict in the Eastern Democratic Republic of Congo, now with some of the highest HIV rates in Africa, cannot be ignored as a contributing factor (Table 19.1).

19.2.7 Food Insecurity and Malnutrition

Food security decreases during conflict for many reasons: destruction of crops and agricultural land, loss of workers, increased prices. The restriction of food in conflict can be considered a weapon of war with 'surrender or starve' tactics documented in conflicts across the middle east, Europe, central Africa and Asia [33, 34].

Table 19.1 Examples of infectious disease outbreaks during conflicts

Cholera	Yemen (2016–2020)
	Dadaab Complex, Kenya (2011, 2015, 2022)
	DRC (recurrent; nationwide 2017)
Diphtheria	Yemen (2017–2019)
	Rohingya refugees in Bangladesh (2017–2019)
Malaria	Afghanistan civil war (1978)
	Tajikistan civil war (1992–1997)
Polio	Sudan (2003)
	Syria (2013)
Typhus	Warsaw Ghetto (1942)
	Auschwitz Concentration Camp (1942–1944)

Food insecurity and the subsequent risk of malnutrition and threat to life is a complex situation, with multi-factorial economic, environmental, political and conflict-related drivers that are interlinked and mutually reinforcing. The exception to this is that of Ukraine, whose current food crisis is almost entirely driven by the 2022 Russian invasion and subsequent economic shocks as it was a relatively food-secure nation prior to this event. Ukraine and the Russian Federation were among the world's most important exporters of grains and fertilisers prior to the war, with a significant proportion of these exports reaching the developing world, with detrimental downstream effects predicted on regions already experiencing food insecurity, sparking a global food crisis [35–37].

Several organisations report on the state of food security across the world. The World Food Programme estimates that 345 million people face high levels of food insecurity in 2023, with 70% of the world's hungry people living in areas affected by conflict and violence. The Integrated Food Insecurity Phase Classification (IPC), produced by the Global Network Against Food Crises, is a system that categorises cases into phases of increasing insecurity, risk of acute malnutrition and threat to life, as well as informing the crisis response to these shortages. The Acute Food Insecurity (AFI) scale has five such phases, with phase 3 representing a crisis requiring urgent action to protect life, livelihood and prevent or revert widespread death. In the 2023 Global Report on Food Crisis, armed conflict and insecurity was a factor driving food insecurity in 26 countries/territories experiencing phase 3 or above AFI, and the most significant driver of acute food insecurity in 19 countries/territories with a cumulative population of 117.1 million people [38]. Whilst these numbers had fallen compared to the 2022 report [39], where 139 million people across 24 countries/territories experienced food insecurity due to conflict, economic shock was a further driver in the 2023 report (27 countries/territories, 83.9 million people). Therefore, armed conflict remains the most important risk factor for food insecurity in terms of total number of people affected.

19.2.8 Childhood Health

The safety and protection of children is a near universal principle that is established in international convention. Article 38 of the United Nations Convention on the Rights of the Child states that governments must 'take all feasible measures to ensure protection and care of children who are affected by an armed conflict' [40]. This convention has been ratified by every member of the United Nations (except for the United States). This article is very important when one considers that nearly 1 in 5 children, roughly 468 million, live in conflict-affected areas [41].

Children are among the most vulnerable groups during war. They not only bear the devastating immediate effects of war: death, injury, sexual assault, they grow up with lasting consequences of psychological damage, disability, poor education and loss of societal structure [42, 43]. These additional burdens contribute to the indirect mortality of conflict. Quantifying the indirect effect of conflict on childhood mortality is difficult, but a review of childhood mortality on the African continent between

1995 and 2015 found that for every direct death from armed conflict, there were at least 3 indirect deaths among children aged 0 to 5 years old [44]. The average life expectancy of children brought up in conflict areas is reduced by as much as 14 years [45].

The impacts of conflict on child health are apparent from birth. Disruption to maternal antenatal care increased maternal stress and food scarcity result in lower birth weights and an increased neonatal morbidity and mortality rates seen in countries affected by war [42, 43, 46]. Food scarcity can make it challenging for parents to provide adequate nutrition, ultimately resulting in malnutrition.

Malnutrition is linked to 45% of deaths in children under 5 years old, and 75% of children who display signs of stunting, a measure of malnutrition affecting child growth, live in conflict-affected areas [47, 48]. The impact of malnutrition in childhood extends into adulthood with increased disease susceptibility, lower educational achievement and decreased adult height and strength [46]. Each of the factors will contribute to the poor health outcomes seen in later life.

Childhood vaccinations are key to reducing many communicable diseases and require a functioning public health system with reliable supply chains and funding to operate. As discussed above, vaccination efforts are affected by conflict. Successful childhood vaccination programmes require a functioning public health system with reliable supply chains and funding to operate [49]. Conflict affects vaccination programmes both directly, such as in conflict-related attacks on vaccination programmes, which occurred in eight countries in 2021 alone [50], and indirectly through healthcare resource redistribution in dealing with the acute pressure of treating the injured [49, 51]. Breakdown in vaccination programmes can result in immediate outbreaks, such as the re-emergence of polio in Syria in 2013, a disease not seen in the country since 1999 [52, 53]. The effect of vaccination schedule disruption is not limited to the period of active conflict. Analysis of the Rubella outbreak in Bosnia and Herzegovina in 2010 found that 43% of cases were among people who had missed out on childhood vaccination during the 3-year war which had ended 15 years prior [42].

The exact number of child soldiers is unknown, but it has been estimated that there are between 250,000 worldwide [54] across seven governmental armed forces and 49 armed groups [55]. These children are exposed to the terrors of war first hand and can suffer into adulthood with mental illness such as posttraumatic stress disorder, and many find it difficult to re-engage in society after war [56].

Case Example: Disrupted Childhood Immunisation During Sierra Leone's Civil War

Between 1991 and 2002, Sierra Leone experienced a nearly 11-year civil war. Development of the country's healthcare system had been poor throughout British Colonial rule, ending in 1961, and this trend continued in the decades post-independence, an era of political unrest and authoritarianism. Despite these challenges, in 1974, The WHO's Expanded Programme of Immunisations (EPI) childhood vaccine schedule was implemented, with rising vaccine coverage and falling childhood mortality up until the onset of the Civil War. Diphtheria/Tetanus/Polio-Pertussis (DPT3) vaccination rates rose from 13% in 1980 to 83% by 1990, and childhood mortality fell from 162.2 per 1000 live births between 1985 and 1987 to 69.9 between 1988 and 1989 [57].

Much of the country's health and economic infrastructure was decimated during the war, with many hospitals ransacked and used as rebel strongholds, or burnt to the ground. During the period of conflict, significant disruption to the EPI vaccine programme occurred, with age-appropriate vaccination rates in children under 3 years old falling to around 55% midway through the conflict. Varying vaccination rates occurred throughout the period of armed conflict, reflecting the differing degree of disruption that periods of more intense conflict resulted in. Children born in Freetown during the Siege of 1997–1998 had significantly lower age-appropriate vaccine rates (as low as 26%) compared to those born in the period of relative calm two years earlier (68%).

Following the war, the healthcare system had to be rebuilt almost entirely from scratch. Vaccination and childhood mortality rates are worse than the pre-war period, and persistent deficits in secondary care exist with low numbers of hospitals and healthcare staff. As of 2008, complete childhood vaccination was only at 40%, and infant mortality was at 89 per 100 live births. The under-five mortality rate at this time was 140 per 1000 [58].

19.3 Armed Conflict and Healthcare Workers

Providing healthcare during conflict is profoundly difficult and places a large burden on healthcare workers. As well as trying to meet the existing healthcare needs, healthcare workers find themselves working in dangerous environments with often limited resources.

Direct violence against healthcare workers has continued to rise, with 1989 incidents in 2022, the highest number of incidents on record [59]. These attacks include 704 healthcare facilities damaged or destroyed, either directly targeted by shelling and looting or indirectly by indiscriminate bombing. The loss of vital health infrastructure severely impairs the ability for care systems to respond to growing health needs during conflict. Some countries have found themselves with almost no hospitals remaining. The 2023 conflict in Sudan has seen its hospital capacity reduced by 70%, from 80 hospitals to only 26 [60]. Fighting can even occur inside hospitals. During a 6-month period (December 2013–June 2014) in the South Sudan conflict, the international healthcare provider Médecins Sans Frontières recorded four separate incidents where medical staff and patients were attacked in hospitals [61]. Over 50 people were killed on hospital grounds. Amid hostilities, healthcare workers

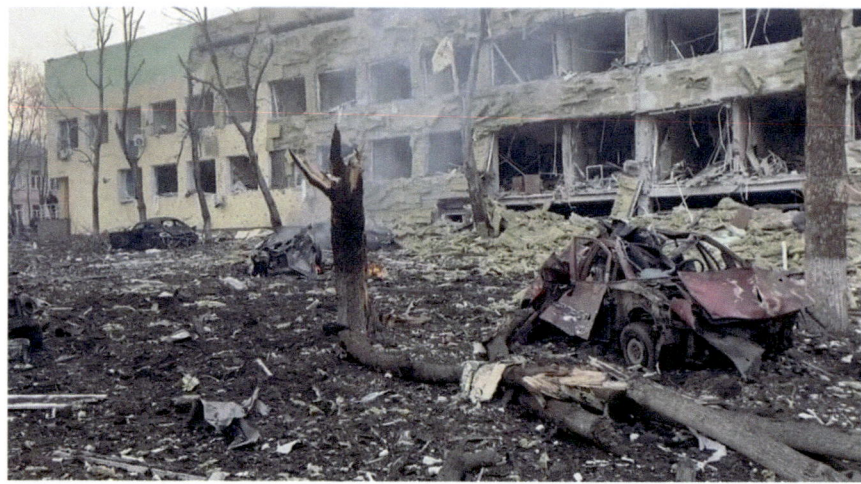

Fig. 19.1 Mariupol's Maternity Hospital No.3 after the airstrike (Courtesy: armyinform.com.ua)

report feeling helpless, unable to provide care for their patients and unable to ensure their own safety [60, 62]. The direct trauma they experience can lead to the development of mental illness, with high levels of anxiety and post-traumatic stress disorder found [62, 63]. The sheer challenge of providing care in such challenging situations also leads to high levels of exhaustion and burnout.

Providing healthcare is therefore extremely costly to the healthcare workers. It is important to remember that healthcare workers are just as vulnerable to conflict and experience the same pressures to flee conflict. This can lead to a skill gap, particularly in the country experiencing conflict. Syria, for example, saw over 50% of its 30,000 doctors leave the country because of the civil war [64]. One of Syria's major cities, Aleppo, went from having 2000 doctors serving a population of over 2 million, to only 40. It is easy to see how countries experiencing conflict struggle to provide healthcare for their population (Fig. 19.1).

19.4   Healthcare of Refugees and Internally Displaced Peoples

As we have discussed, living in conflict-affected areas has health consequences. This impact is carried with groups who flee conflict zones, becoming displaced peoples [64]. Two groups emerge, internally displaced people (IDPs) and refugees. A refugee can be defined as a person forced to flee their country because of violence or persecution. Refugees benefit from international treaties that protect their rights to seek asylum and access healthcare. IDPs, like refugees in that they have been forced to flee, have not crossed their state border, and therefore do not benefit from the same protections as refugees [65]. Regardless of where they are displaced, both experience profound health impacts.

Both groups may move to existing urban centres or to established camps [63]. Urban centres can benefit from established healthcare infrastructure, such as facilities, diagnostics and healthcare workers. Camps face the challenge of having to develop health structures from scratch. This is a situation familiar to humanitarian organisations, who may find it difficult to integrate into local health services [64 , 66, 67]. However, both settings are vulnerable to being under-resourced. Scaling up services requires financial and human resources, which can be challenging to source and protect when there is nearby conflict.

The movement of refugees and IDPs causes rapid increases in populations and often results in poor housing provision with limited sanitation. This results in the rapid transmission of transmittable diseases. As we have already established, conflict-affected communities have lower vaccination rates so are particularly vulnerable during disease outbreaks [64].

Both groups of displaced people often flee with little time to prepare. Healthcare records are left behind or lost in the attacks on facilities. This profoundly impacts those with chronic non- communicable diseases. They struggle to receive the medications and follow-up needed, impeding their long-term health outcomes, and resulting in higher indirect mortality [68].

Refugees may face the additional barriers of linguistic and cultural differences when trying to access healthcare [64, 66]. The country of refuge may not provide equivalent free healthcare services, which might mean that individuals aren't able to afford more than rudimentary healthcare, or only be able to access care that is being provided by humanitarian relief organisations. Countries can also structure services in a different way, which can prevent refugees from accessing healthcare in accordance with their needs.

19.5 Humanitarian Assistance in Conflict Zones

The objectives of humanitarian action are to save lives, alleviate suffering and maintain dignity during periods of crisis, man-made or natural. Numerous organisations are involved in the provision of aid to those affected by armed conflict, the most recognisable likely being the International Committee of the Red Cross, founded in 1863 (see Fig. 19.2) and given a mandate by Geneva Convention signatories to protect victims of armed conflict, and Médecins Sans Frontières.

In 1965 at the 20th International Conference of the Red Cross, a series of fundamental principles were proclaimed, guiding the ethical and operational actions of the movement [69]:

1. Humanity—prevent and alleviate suffering, protect life and health, and respect for the human being
2. Impartiality—action without discrimination

Fig. 19.2 Henry Dunant:
Founder of the
International Committee of
the Red Cross (1863)

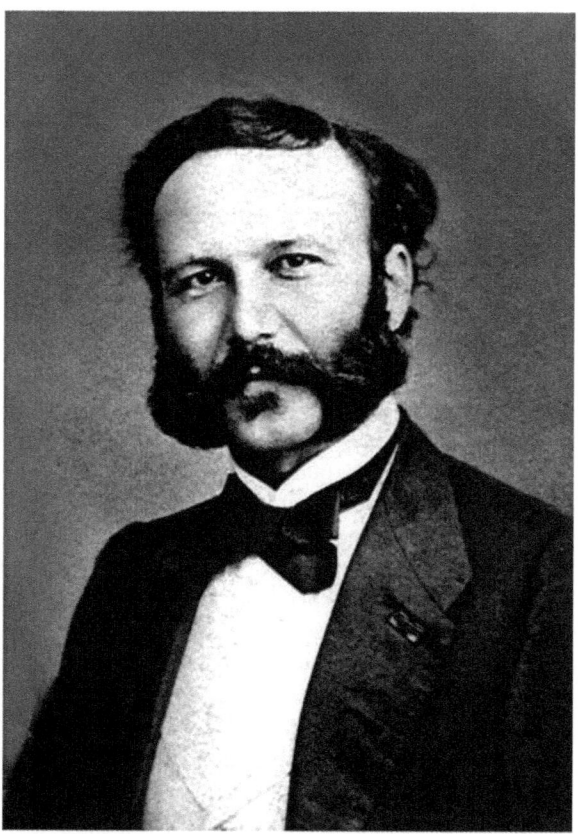

3. Independence—independent from political, economic, military, or other humanitarian objectives
4. Neutrality—abstain from taking sides or engaging in debate and controversy.

Voluntary service, unity and universality were three further principles established at this conference; however, it is the first four that have been adopted by
organisations worldwide.

19.6   Barriers to Humanitarian Aid

There are four major constraints on the provision of humanitarian assistance in
armed conflict zones [70]:

1. Violence and insecurity
2. Bureaucratic constraints
3. Counter-terrorism regulations
4. Funding

Every year, over 150 aid workers are wounded or kidnapped, and over 50 killed, the overwhelming majority, over 90%, being local aid workers. Organisations may become the target of armed groups during the theft of aid resources, and security for the delivery of relief brings with it financial pressures.

Visa denial or delay, as well as imposing taxation and fees on the import of relief items and equipment by the State in which an organisation is trying to conduct their activities within can hamper their operations. In 2017, visa delays posed challenges in the delivery of aid to the Rohingya peoples in Myanmar by overseas aid professionals, and in South Sudan, fees were raised to $10,000 for humanitarian personnel in that same year. Organisations need to be mindful of working in regions with sanctioned terrorist groups, as their activity may be deemed to be supportive of these groups and could therefore face prosecution under counter-terrorism legislation.

> **Case Example: The Death of Aid Worker Peter Kassig**
>
> Peter Kassig was an American humanitarian worker, aiding Syrian refugees in Syria and Lebanon in 2012. Initially working as a medical assistant in a Lebanese hospital treating refugees fleeing the Syrian Civil War, ongoing to this day since 2011, he founded the organisation Special Emergency Response and Assistance (SERA) providing refugees with medical aid and supplies, clothing and food.
>
> Whilst en route to deliver aid, food and supplies to refugees in eastern Syria in October 2013, Kassig was kidnapped by the Islamic State of Iraq and the Levant (ISIL) and held with journalists Nicolas Hénin and John Cantlie. Following the execution of Alan Henning, an English humanitarian aid worker, in an ISIL released video, Kassig was named as the next victim to be beheaded and was revealed to have been executed in a video in November 2014.
>
> Alongside Peter Kassig, over 60 kidnappings of aid workers occurred in 2013 and 120 killings in 2014. Humanitarian Outcomes, an organisation conducting research into humanitarian aid, publishes the Aid Worker Security Database that reports on the deliberate acts of violence against aid workers. There has been an overall trend of an increasing number of attacks and victims, following a brief decline in 2013, and the indiscriminate use of airstrikes during the 2022 Russian invasion of Ukraine threatens to push these figures higher.

References

1. International Committee of the Red Cross. How is the Term "Armed Conflict" Defined in International Humanitarian Law? 2008. Available from: https://www.icrc.org/en/doc/resources/documents/article/other/armed-conflict-article-170308.htm
2. Kaldor M. New and old wars: organized violence in a global era. 3rd ed. Cambridge: Polity; 2013.
3. Otterbein KF, Ebrary I. How war began. College Station: Texas A&M University Press; 2004.

4. Burkle FM. Revisiting the battle of Solferino: the worsening plight of civilian casualties in war and conflict. Dis Med Public Health Preparedness. 2019;13(5–6):837–41.

5. Ghobarah HA, Huth P, Russett B. Civil wars kill and maim people—long after the shooting stops. Am Polit Sci Rev. 2003;97(02):189–202.

6. Krause K. From armed conflict to political violence: mapping & explaining conflict trends. Daedalus. 2016;145(4):113–26.

7. 'War's Greatest Cost Is Its Human Toll', Secretary-General Reminds Peacebuilding Commission, Warning of 'Perilous Impunity' Taking Hold [press release]. United Nations Press. 2022.

8. Brubaker R, Day A, Huvé S. COVID-19 and humanitarian access: how the pandemic should provoke systemic change in the global humanitarian system. United Nations University; 2021 Apr 6.

9. Sartin JS. Infectious diseases during the Civil War: the triump of the "Third Army". Clin Infect Dis. 1993;16(4):580–4.

10. Burki T. The illustrious dead: the terrifying story of how typhus killed Napoleon's greatest army. Lancet Inf Dis. 2010;10(11):748.

11. Hyams KC, Hanson K, Stephen Wignall F, Escamilla J, Oldfield EC. The impact of infectious diseases on the health of U.S. Troops deployed to the Persian Gulf during operations desert shield and desert storm. Clin Inf Dis. 1995;20(6):1497–504.

12. Letendre K, Fincher CL, Thornhill R. Does infectious disease cause global variation in the frequency of intrastate armed conflict and civil war? Bio Rev. 2010;85(3):669–83.

13. Ember CR, Ember M. Resource unpredictability, mistrust, and war. J Conf Resol. 1992;36(2):242–62.

14. Morris-Iverson L, Granillo E, Grundin S. Water under fire: attacks on water and sanitation services in armed conflict and the impact on children. 2021 May [accessed 2023 Jul 11]. Available from: https://www.unicef.org/reports/water-under-fire-volume-3

15. Dureab FA, Shibib K, Al-Yousufi R, Jahn A. Yemen: Cholera outbreak and the ongoing armed conflict. J Inf Devel Countries. 2018;12(05):397–403.

16. Charnley GEC, Jean K, Kelman I, Gaythorpe KAM, Murray KA. Association between conflict and cholera in Nigeria and the democratic Republic of the Congo. Emerg Inf Dis. 2022;28(12):2472–81.

17. Ingelbeen B, Hendrickx D, Miwanda B, van der MAB S, Mossoko M, Vochten H, et al. Recurrent cholera outbreaks, democratic Republic of the Congo, 2008–2017. Emerg Inf Dis. 2019;25(5):856–64.

18. Elyajouri A, Abilkacem R, Agadr A. Report on paediatric care in the Moroccan military mission in the Gaza Strip. Eastern Mediterranean Health J. 2017;23(11):781–5.

19. Golicha Q, Shetty S, Nasiblov O, Hussein A, Wainaina E, Obonyo M, et al. Cholera outbreak in Dadaab Refugee Camp, Kenya — November 2015–June 2016. MMWR Morb Mortal Weekly Rep. 2018;67(34):958–61.

20. United Nations. Cholera outbreak hits Kenya's largest refugee complex – UN agency. 2011. Available from: https://news.un.org/en/story/2011/11/394962

21. UNICEF. Kenya Humanitarian Situation Report. 2018 Dec [accessed 11 July 2023]. Available from: https://www.unicef.org/media/74961/file/Kenya-SitRep-December-2018.pdf

22. UNICEF. Humanitarian Situation Report No. 5 Kenya. 2023 Jul [accessed 11 July 2023]. Available from: https://www.unicef.org/media/142666/file/UNICEF%20Kenya%20 Humanitarian%20Situation%20Report%20No.%205,%201%20-%2031%20May%20 2023.pdf

23. Rahman MR, Islam K. Massive diphtheria outbreak among Rohingya refugees: lessons learnt. J Travel Med. 2019;26(1) https://doi.org/10.1093/jtm/tay122.

24. Polonsky JA, Ivey M, Mazhar MdKA, Rahman Z, le Polain de Waroux O, Karo B, et al. Epidemiological, clinical, and public health response characteristics of a large outbreak of diphtheria among the Rohingya population in Cox's Bazar, Bangladesh, 2017 to 2019: a retrospective study. Spiegel P, editor. PLOS Medicine. 2021 Apr 1;18(4):e1003587.

25. Dureab F, Al-Sakkaf M, Ismail O, Kuunibe N, Krisam J, Müller O, et al. Diphtheria outbreak in Yemen: the impact of conflict on a fragile health system. Conflict and Health. 2019 ;13(1).
26. van Pelt RJ. The case for Auschwitz: evidence from the irving trial. Bloomington: Indiana University Press; 2002.
27. Stone L, He D, Lehnstaedt S, Artzy-Randrup Y. Extraordinary curtailment of massive typhus epidemic in the Warsaw Ghetto. Science. Advances. 2020;6(30):eabc0927.
28. Gayer M, Legros D, Formenty P, Connolly MA. Conflict and emerging infectious diseases. Emerg Inf Dis. 2007;13(11):1625–31.
29. Wells CR, Pandey A, Ndeffo Mbah ML, Bernard-A G, Malvy D, Singer BH, et al. The exacerbation of Ebola outbreaks by conflict in the Democratic Republic of the Congo. Proc Nat Acad Sci. 2019;116(48):24633–373.
30. Gele AA, Bjune GA. Armed conflicts have an impact on the spread of tuberculosis: the case of the Somali Regional State of Ethiopia. Conf Health. 2010;4(1). https://doi.org/10.1186/1752-1505-4-1.
31. Akil L, Ahmad HA. The recent outbreaks and reemergence of poliovirus in war and conflict-affected areas. Int J Inf Dis. 2016;49:40–6.
32. Ottolini MG, Cirks BT, Madden KB, Rajnik M. Pediatric infectious diseases encountered during wartime—Part 1: experiences and lessons learned from armed conflict in the modern era. 2021 Dec 1;23(12).
33. Global Rights Compliance. Starvation case studies archives. 2022 [accessed 10 July 2023]. Available from: https://starvationaccountability.org/content/starvation-case-study/
34. Conley B, de Waal A. The purposes of starvation: historical and contemporary uses. J Int Crim Jus. 2019;17(4):699–722. https://doi.org/10.1093/jicj/mqz054.
35. Food and Agricultural Organisation of the United Nations. Ukraine: impact of the war on agricultural enterprises – findings of a nationwide survey of agricultural enterprises with land up to 250 hectares, January-February 2023. 2023 [accessed 11 July 2023]. Available from: https://www.fao.org/documents/card/en?details=CC5755EN
36. Food and Agricultural Organisation of the United Nations. The importance of Ukraine and the Russian federation for global agricultural markets and the risks associated with the war in Ukraine. 2022 [accessed 11 July 2023]. Available from: https://www.fao.org/3/cb9013en/cb9013en.pdf
37. Nguyen TT, Timilsina RR, Sonobe T, Rahut DB. Interstate war and food security: implications from Russia's invasion of Ukraine. Front Sust Food Syst. 2023:7. https://doi.org/10.3389/fsufs.2023.1080696.
38. World Food Programme. The Global Report on Food Crises 2023. 2023 May [accessed 11 July 2023]. Available from: https://www.wfp.org/publications/global-report-food-crises-2023
39. World Food Programme. Global Report on Food Crises – 2022. 2022 May [accessed 11 July 2023]. Available from: https://www.wfp.org/publications/global-report-food-crises-2022
40. United Nations. Convention on the rights of the child (1989) Treaty no. 27531. United Nations Treaty Series, 1577, pp. 3–178. [accessed 8 July 2023] Available from: https://treaties.un.org/doc/Treaties/1990/09/19900902%2003-14%20AM/Ch_IV_11p.pdf
41. Save the Children. Children In Conflict. 2023 [accessed 13 July 2023]. Available from: https://data.stopwaronchildren.org/
42. Jawad M, Hone T, Vamos EP, Cetorelli V, Millett C. Implications of armed conflict for maternal and child health: a regression analysis of data from 181 countries for 2000–2019. PLOS Med. 2021;18(9) https://doi.org/10.1371/journal.pmed.1003810.
43. Barbara JS. The impact of war on children and imperative to end war. Croatian J Med. 2006;47(6):891–4.
44. Wagner Z, Heft-Neal S, Bhutta ZA, Black RE, Burke M, Bendavid E. Armed conflict and child mortality in Africa: a geospatial analysis. Lancet. 2018;392(10150):857–65. https://doi.org/10.1016/s0140-6736(18)31437-5.

45. Aburto JM, di Lego V, Riffe T, Kashyap R, van Raalte A, Torrisi O. A global assessment of the impact of violence on lifetime uncertainty. Science Advances. 2023 Feb 3 [accessed 8 July 2023];9(5). https://doi.org/10.1126/sciadv.add9038.

46. Martins VJ, Toledo Florêncio TM, Grillo LP, Do CP, Franco M, Martins PA, Clemente AP, et al. Long-lasting effects of undernutrition. Int J Envir Res Public Health. 2011;8(6):1817–46. https://doi.org/10.3390/ijerph8061817.

47. World Health Organization. Fact sheets – malnutrition. 2021 [accessed 10 July 2023]. Available from: https://www.who.int/news-room/fact-sheets/detail/malnutrition

48. World Food Programme. Hunger and Conflict fact sheet. 2018 [accessed 10 July 2023]. Available from: https://www.wfp.org/publications/hunger-and-conflict-fact-sheet-2018

49. Obradovic Z, Balta S, Obradovic A, Mesic S. The impact of war on vaccine preventable diseases. Materia Socio Medica. 2014;26(6):382. https://doi.org/10.5455/msm.2014.26.382-384.

50. Insecurity Insights. Attacked and threatened: health care at risk. 2023 [accessed 10 July 2023]. Available from: https://map.insecurityinsight.org/health

51. DeLand K. Vaccine equity in conflict-affected areas: the challenges of development, production, procurement, and Distribution. 2022 [accessed 10 July 2023]. Available from: https://www.ipinst.org/2022/05/vaccine-equity-in-conflict-affected-areas-the-challenges-of-development-production-procurement-and-distribution

52. Ahmad B, Bhattacharya S. Polio eradication in Syria. Lancet Inf Dis. 2014;14(7):547–8. https://doi.org/10.1016/s1473-3099(14)70803-5.

53. Al-Moujahed A, Alahdab F, Abolaban H, Beletsky L. Polio in Syria: problem still not solved. Avicenna J Med. 2017;7(2):64–6. https://doi.org/10.4103/ajm.AJM_173_16.

54. Peace Direct. Child soldiers – Peace direct. 2019 [accessed 11 July 2023]. Available from: https://www.peacedirect.org/child-soldiers/

55. UNICEF. Ending the recruitment and use of children in armed conflict. 2015 [accessed 11 July 2023]. Available from: https://www.unicef.org.uk/publications/child-soldiers-briefing/

56. Boothby N, Rosenfield A, Nichol B. Child soldiering: impact on childhood development and learning capacity. Protect Education in Insecurity and Conflict (PEIC); 2010 Jan. Available at: https://inee.org/sites/default/files/resources/Boothby-Impact_on_Learning.pdf

57. Senessie C, Gage GN, von Elm E. Delays in childhood immunization in a conflict area: a study from Sierra Leone during civil war. Conf Health. 2007;1(1):14.

58. Statistics Sierra Leone and ICF Macro. Sierra Leone Demographic and Health Survey 2008: Key Findings. 2009 [accessed 11 July 2023]. Available from: https://dhsprogram.com/pubs/pdf/SR171/SR171.pdf

59. Safeguarding Health in Conflict Coalition. Ignoring Red Lines: Violence Against Health Care in Conflict 2022. Safeguarding Health in Conflict Coalition; 2023.

60. USAID. Attacks on health workers and facilities worsen a dire humanitarian situation in Sudan. 2023 [accessed 12 July 2023]. Available from: https://www.usaid.gov/news-information/press-releases/may-04-2023-attacks-health-workers-and-facilities-worsen-dire-humanitarian-situation-sudan

61. MSF. South Sudan conflict: Violence against healthcare. 2014 [accessed 12 July 2023]. Available from: https://www.msf.org/sites/default/files/2018-06/msf-south_sudan_conflict-violence_against_healthcare%202014.pdf

62. Shamia NA, Thabet AA, Vostanis P. Exposure to war traumatic experiences, post-traumatic stress disorder and post-traumatic growth among nurses in Gaza. J Psychiat Mental Health Nur. 2015;22(10):749–55. https://doi.org/10.1111/jpm.12264.

63. Kondrat A. How Russia destroyed the healthcare sector in Mariupol: report by the Ukrainian Healthcare Center (Uhc). Bondar Y, editor. 2023 Jan [accessed 11 July 2023]. Available from: https://uhc.org.ua/en/2023/01/04/healthcare-in-mariupol/

64. Alhaffar MH, Janos S. Public health consequences after ten years of the Syrian crisis: a literature review. Global Health. 2021;17(1). https://doi.org/10.1186/s12992-021-00762-9.

65. PHR. Syria's Medical Community Under Assault. Physicians for Human Rights; 2014 [accessed 12 July 2023]. Available from: https://s3.amazonaws.com/PHR_other/Syria%27s-Medical-Community-Under-Assault-October-2014.pdf
66. Ojeleke O, Groot W, Pavlova M. Care delivery among refugees and internally displaced persons affected by complex emergencies: a systematic review of the literature. J Public Health. 2020;30(3):747–62. https://doi.org/10.1007/s10389-020-01343-7.
67. UNHCR. Handbook for Emergencies. 3rd ed. The office of the United Nations High Commissioner for Refugees (UNHCR); 2007.
68. Idris I. Effectiveness of various refugee settlement approaches. K4D Helpdesk Report 223 Brighton, United Kingdom: Institute for Development Studies; 2017.
69. International Committee of the Red Cross. Fundamental Principles of the Red Cross and Red Crescent Movement. 2016 [accessed 11 July 2023]. Available from: https://www.icrc.org/en/document/fundamental-principles-red-cross-and-red-crescent
70. Kurtzer J. Never More Necessary: Overcoming Humanitarian Access Challenges [Internet]. Centre for Strategic International Studies; 2019 Sep [accessed 11 July 2023]. Available from: https://www.csis.org/analysis/never-more-necessary-overcoming-humanitarian-access-challenges#h2-types-of-access-constraints-

Bibliography

Doctors without borders | The Practical Guide to Humanitarian Law [Internet]. Medicine Sans Frontieres. 2010 [cited 2023 Jul 11]. Available from: https://guide-humanitarian-law.org/content/article/3/international-armed-conflict-iac/
International Committee of the Red Cross. War & Law [Internet]. War & Law | International Committee of the Red Cross. 2019 [cited 2023 Jul 11]. Available from: https://www.icrc.org/en/war-and-law
IPC Global Partners. 2021. Integrated food security phase classification technical manual version 3.1. Evidence and standards for better food security and nutrition decisions. Rome. Available from: https://www.ipcinfo.org/fileadmin/user_upload/ipcinfo/manual/IPC_Technical_Manual_3_Final.pdf
Roser M, Hasell J, Herre B, Macdonald B. War and peace [Internet]. Our World in Data. 2016 [cited 2023 Jul 11]. Available from: https://ourworldindata.org/war-and-peace
The Rule of Law in Armed Conflict Project | RULAC [Internet]. Rule of Law in Armed Conflicts. Geneva Academy; [cited 2023 Jul 11]. Available from: https://www.rulac.org/
Treaties, States Parties and Commentaries database [Internet]. IHL Treaties. International Committee of the Red Cross; 2022 [cited 2023 Jul 11]. Available from: https://ihl-databases.icrc.org/en/ihl-treaties
UNHCR. Ukraine Refugee Situation [Internet]. Operational Data Portal | Ukraine Refugee Situation. UNHCR; 2022. Available from: https://data.unhcr.org/en/situations/ukraine

Chapter 20
Humanitarian Aid

Catrin Kruppa, William Harman-Cashmore, and Lizzie O'Brien

20.1 Humanitarian Aid

20.1.1 What Is Humanitarian Aid?

Humanitarian aid delivers lifesaving, needs-based assistance to people affected by human-made and natural disasters. Support is offered impartially, regardless of gender, race, nationality, political or religious beliefs. Those in need of humanitarian aid include refugees, homeless people, victims of war, natural disasters and famine. In 2019, 168 million people needed humanitarian assistance [1].

20.1.2 Principles of Humanitarian Aid

The Office for the Coordination of Humanitarian Aid describes the four Principles of Humanitarian Aid, based upon International Humanitarian Law. These principles are the foundations for humanitarian assistance: [2]

- *Humanity:* human suffering must be addressed wherever present
- *Neutrality:* aid must not favour any side in conflict
- *Impartiality:* aid must be provided solely based on need, without discrimination
- *Independence:* autonomy of humanitarian objectives from political, economic, military or other objectives.

C. Kruppa · W. Harman-Cashmore · L. O'Brien (✉)
School of Medicine, Cardiff University, Cardiff, UK
e-mail: kruppac@cardiff.ac.uk; harman-cashmorew@cardiff.ac.uk; obrienl9@cardiff.ac.uk

A. Fiander, G. Fry (eds.), *A Healthcare Students Introduction to Global Health*,
https://doi.org/10.1007/978-3-031-66563-9_20

20.1.3   Humanitarian Law

Humanitarian law underpins humanitarian aid, aiming to limit the effects of armed conflict on civilians. It states responsibilities that all groups involved in conflict must follow, including the rapid and unimpeded passage of humanitarian relief, freedom of movement of humanitarian personnel and protection of civilians, refugees, prisoners, wounded and the sick. Where Humanitarian Law is violated, civilian and humanitarian workers' lives are at risk [3].

20.1.4   Who Is Involved in Humanitarian Aid?

Humanitarian aid is delivered by both international bodies and non-governmental organisations (NGOs), a snapshot of which are described below:

20.1.5   The United Nations (UN) [4]

The Office for the Coordination of Humanitarian Affairs (OCHA) coordinates the UN's response to emergencies and humanitarian crises. Different entities include:

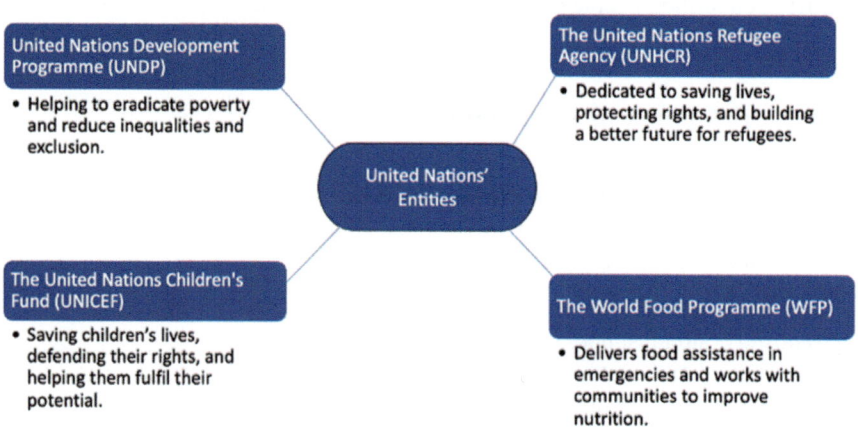

20.1.6   The World Health Organisation (WHO) [5]

The WHO works to prevent health emergencies and support the development of tools that are needed during outbreaks, respond to acute health emergencies and deliver essential health services. During disasters and displacement of people, the

WHO delivers medical services such as routine immunisations, surgical care and treatment for non-communicable diseases [6].

20.1.7   International Federation of Red Cross and Red Crescent Societies (IFRC) [7]

The IFRC is the world's largest humanitarian and development network. It provides international assistance without discrimination following natural and human-made disasters.

20.1.8   Médecins Sans Frontières (MSF) [8]

An NGO delivering emergency medical assistance to people affected by armed conflict, epidemics, pandemics, natural disasters and exclusion from healthcare.

20.1.9   Case Study: Yemen in Crisis [9]

Yemen hosts one of the largest humanitarian crises in the world, with over 21 million people in need of humanitarian aid. The conflict escalated in 2015 and has caused more than 12,000 civilian deaths. Yemen imported 90% of its food before the conflict, and the flow has been massively disrupted. Now, 70% of the population suffer from food insecurity and malnutrition, and 10 million people face famine. *Oxfam* have supplied clean water and sanitation services and provided families with money to buy food or livestock in the local market, as well as set up cash for work programmes to provide a source of income.

20.1.10   When Is Humanitarian Aid Needed?

Aid may be needed for many reasons and in any country. The need for humanitarian aid is a balance between the severity of the harm ensued and the affected country's capacity to mitigate the impact of a crisis.

In cases of large-scale disasters, even the most well-equipped countries may struggle to support their populations and must rely on humanitarian aid, for example the earthquake and tsunami in Japan in 2011. Alternatively, where a country lacks sufficient resources to begin with, disasters can exacerbate existing challenges within the country, and in some cases, there may be no precipitating physical disaster, rather, a country requires humanitarian aid due economic or governance issues.

Humanitarian aid is needed with disproportionate frequency amongst low-resource countries (LRCs) [10]. This is in part due to reduced infrastructure within LRCs to prevent or mitigate disasters, meaning smaller scale disasters such as low magnitude earthquakes or brief droughts have a much larger impact than in high-resource settings. Additionally, LRCs have a higher incidence of conflict and natural disasters, due to a complex range of factors, including historical global inequity and geographical location in vulnerable places [11].

20.1.11   Natural Disasters

Natural disasters come in many different forms with varied and severe effects. Examples include earthquakes, tsunamis, volcanic eruptions, floods and drought, many of which are on the increase with climate change.

Loss of life occurs through a variety of means, both immediately and in the longer term. For example, destructive events such as earthquakes and tsunamis pose immediate threat to life via building collapse or directly from the disaster itself (e.g. drowning), whilst loss of infrastructure and economy result in poverty, political unrest and poor health outcomes in the longer term.

This loss of life is exacerbated in LRCs for several reasons:

- Houses in LRCs are more likely to be self-built and may not adhere to the rigorous building standards required to withstand disasters such as an earthquake or landslide. Buildings may also be based in more vulnerable locations, like a hillside.
- LRCs often have limited infrastructure, and so resources such as public services may be less resistant to disruption or increased demand. Minimal facilities also impede aid efforts, for example, if roads and transport links are limited, delivering aid to more remote locations is difficult.
- A reduced availability of quality healthcare also increases the loss of life, not just in management of initial injuries, but also in preventing and managing more chronic conditions, such as resulting disability. Population health may also be poor due to reduced health coverage and access in LRCs, meaning populations are more vulnerable to health threats, such as infectious diseases spreading when unvaccinated populations are brought together following disasters. Health outcomes are further worsened by any damage to infrastructure as medical supplies and personnel become scarce.
- LRCs often suffer from economic and political instability due to resource scarcity, which can result in increased rates of crime, unemployment and poverty. These in turn impact on health status, for example injury or loss of life due to violence.

20.1.12   Case Study: Haiti Earthquake 2010 [12]

In 2010, a 7.0 magnitude earthquake struck Haiti, an island nation. It resulted in the death of 200,000 people, and over 2 million people were left homeless. Due to poor quality buildings and infrastructure, attributed to a struggling economy, there was large-scale destruction and trauma resulting from building collapse. The loss of infrastructure made getting aid to the affected areas difficult. This exacerbated the crisis, and Haiti needed support from governments and NGOs. In this case, the country received support from countries such as Cuba and NGOs including MSF.

20.1.13   Conflict

Conflict often occurs in LRCs; largely due to historical injustices of wealth and power globally, and where conflict occurs, it plunges countries into further scarcity. As with natural disasters, the effects of conflict not only result in an increase of trauma injuries, but also the loss of infrastructure that results in more medium- to long-term impact.

The differences arise due to the period that conflicts can occur. The trauma injuries being the result of a natural disaster occur in a narrow window, whilst trauma injuries because of conflict occur for the duration of that conflict, especially in more modern times as the burden of war is shifted more onto civilians.

This idea of time is also important when considering supply lines and infrastructure. In war, if a road is cut off, it is typically done so deliberately, to besiege a city or cut off supplies to enemies. This means that unlike in natural disasters, the infrastructure remains destroyed for as long as whoever is blocking or destroying it remains there. Therefore, the main difference is that impact on civilians is intentional.

Humanitarian aid is not just about materials, but also logistical support and skills. Often in conflict, skilled professionals leave the affected area, having the financial capacity and necessary connections to make the journey. This means that the quality of systems like healthcare and public services is greatly diminished and requires humanitarian aid in the form of healthcare professionals being brought in from other countries, like the role of MSF for example.

20.2   Displacement

20.2.1   What Is Displacement?

A displaced person is someone who has had to leave their home due to conflict, violence, human rights violations or natural or human-made disasters [13].

Displacement is sadly not a rare occurrence, and by the end of 2019, 79.5 million people needed protection and assistance because of forced displacement, half of these being children. This is equivalent to 1 person becoming displaced every 2 seconds—roughly 15 people in the time taken to read this paragraph [14].

20.2.2 Where Do People Go?

Displaced people face a limited choice of where to move; either moving elsewhere within their country (internally displaced people) or leaving the country completely, usually entering neighbouring countries, becoming 'refugees' and 'asylum seekers' [13].

Just 16% of the world's refugees are hosted by high-resource countries, placing the responsibility of refugee welfare disproportionately on those who can least afford it [15]. Being low- and middle- income countries themselves, neighbouring, host countries often have limited means to support existing populations, let alone the additional numbers of displaced people.

Humanitarian aid is therefore crucial to support refugees when the host countries often lack the capacity to do so (Fig. 20.1).

20.2.3 Dignity and Displacement

Ensuring aid is dignified is crucial to its success; dignified aid promotes self-esteem and confidence which is so often lacking amongst displaced people and is accordingly listed amongst the Sphere Project's key principles [17]. Dignity is crucial to quality of life, and whilst it can be easily overlooked in the face of life-threatening disaster, it is imperative to remember having a reason to live is just as important as the means to live. Furthermore, using relief efforts that promote dignity also improves the outcomes of aid offered.

20.2.4 Sphere Handbook [18]

The Sphere project is an initiative developed by several NGOs and sets out a rights-based framework for humanitarian aid. Its principles are written in the Humanitarian Charter, which are as follows:

- the right to life with dignity
- the right to receive humanitarian assistance
- the right to protection and security.

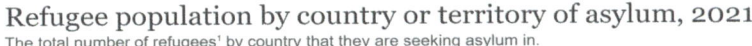

Refugee population by country or territory of asylum, 2021
The total number of refugees¹ by country that they are seeking asylum in.

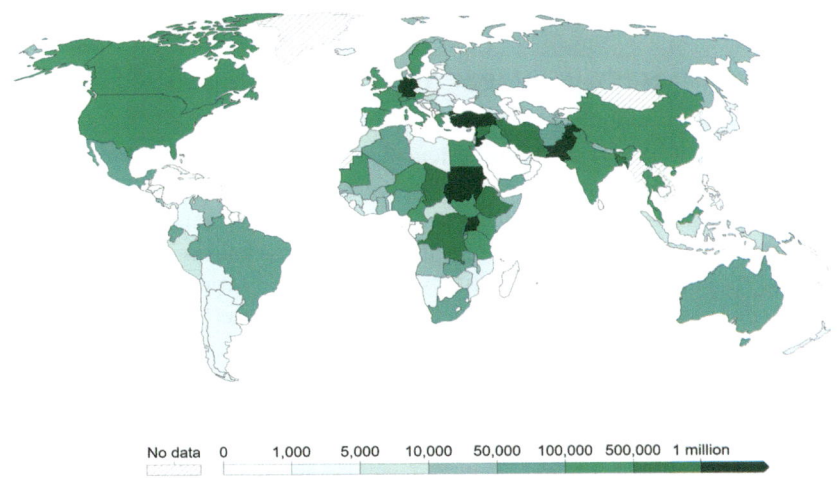

No data   0   1,000   5,000   10,000   50,000   100,000 500,000 1 million

Fig. 20.1 Refugee population by country or territory of asylum, 2021 [16]

20.2.5   *What Is Dignity?*

Dignity is understood as an 'umbrella term' which includes many key components [17]. Interestingly, exactly what these components are varies amongst different refugee communities, who each hold different perceptions of dignity.

The two most identified themes include self-sufficiency and respect, recognising the former facilitates the ability to provide for oneself and family, without the reliance on others, whilst respect of both culture and identity is a critical component of dignity. Other themes addressed include safety, pride, honour (of the individual, family and culture), autonomy of decisions and ownership of possession or land.

In the context of humanitarian aid, these features take different forms, such as the provision of cash rather than food packages (thereby affording individuals the choice and control over what to eat) or, for example, providing religious clothing as essential items (therefore affording women the ability to go out in public).

Communication is key to facilitating an individual's involvement in aid and sustaining a sense of control in what is already a deeply distressing time. There is a keen focus on face-to-face communication over alternative methods such as text, as this avoids barriers such as illiteracy and phone access. Strong communication methods promote inclusion, improving the overall efficacy of aid and relations between workers and refugees.

As summarised by Oxely [19]:

'Whilst *what* a humanitarian agency does in terms of meeting the basic needs of disaster victims is essential to sustain lives, *how* it does this is fundamental to maintaining human dignity'.

Measures to promote dignity often require little time or money but result in profound impact on the efficacy of aid delivered.

20.2.6 Case Study: Rohingya Refugees in Bangladesh [20]

The government of Myanmar has systematically persecuted the Rohingya, a predominantly Muslim ethnic minority in the country, by denying basic rights and targeting them with military campaigns. The hostility has existed for years but culminated more recently in the government's latest crackdown in 2017, following previous violent attacks on the Rohingya community. Fearing for their lives and culture, millions fled across the border to Bangladesh where they live in refugee camps and rely on humanitarian aid. Many of the community have lived in the camps for over ten years and continue to do so whilst the crisis evolves.

The perception of dignity in the camps has been mixed, often stemming from cultural and religious misunderstandings. For example, many women felt uncomfortable receiving their 'dignity packs' of sanitary products whilst queuing alongside men, especially as religious beliefs often require gender segregation in particular circumstances. Furthermore, the packs included a white cloth which for the Rohingya people is a symbolic piece used in funerals. Having witnessed so much death during the escape of Myanmar, the provision of these white cloths was a stark and insensitive reminder of the pain many had endured. Poor communication from aid workers also left many refugees confused, for example, over how allocations of resources were decided. Living in so much confusion compounded the refugees' sense of indignity by reiterating the lack of control in their lives [17].

Solutions Promoting dignity often requires simple and inexpensive solutions, such as:

- a greater understanding of local culture obtained through engaging with professionals like anthropologists. In this example, a better cultural appreciation led to replacing the white cloths in the 'dignity packs' for a more appropriate substitute.
- improved communication between those giving and receiving aid. In this case, clarifying with the refugees how resources were allocated would prevent confusion and empower refugees with the knowledge of how aid was provided.

These solutions have the potential to improve relationships and overall delivery of aid.

References

1. UNICEF. Global annual results report 2019: Humanitarian action. New York: UNICEF; 2020.
2. European Commission. Humanitarian Principals. 2020 [accessed 11 November 2020]. Available from: https://civil-protection-humanitarian-aid.ec.europa.eu/who/humanitarian-

principles_en#:~:text=The%20principles%20of%20humanity%2C%20neutrality,are%20 fundamental%20to%20humanitarian%20action

3. European Commission. International Humanitarian Law. 2020 [accessed 11 November 2020]. Available from: https://ec.europa.eu/echo/what/humanitarian-aid/ international-humanitarian-law_en

4. United Nations. Deliver humanitarian aid. 2020 [accessed 11 November 2020]. Available from: https://www.un.org/en/our-work/deliver-humanitarian-aid

5. World Health Organisation. What we do. 2020 [accessed 11 November 2020]. Available from: https://www.who.int/about/what-we-do

6. World Health Organisation Department for Emergency Risk Management and Humanitarian Response. 2015 WHO humanitarian response. 2015 [accessed 11 November 2020]. Available from: https://www.who.int/hac/who_humanitarian_response_plans2015.pdf?ua=1

7. International Federation of Red Cross and Red Crescent Societies. About the IFRC. 2023 [accessed 3 June 2023]. Available from: https://www.ifrc.org/who-we-are/about-ifrc

8. Médecins Sans Frontières: Who we are. 2020 [accessed 11 November 2020]. Available from: https://www.msf.org/who-we-are

9. Oxfam. Crisis in Yemen. 2020 [accessed 12 November 2020]. Available from: https://www. oxfam.org/en/what-we-do/emergencies/crisis-yemen

10. Urquhart A, Girling-Morris F, Mason E, Nelson-Pollard S. Global Humanitarian Assistance Report 2023. UK: Development Initiatives; 2023. Available from: https://devinit.org/resources/ global-humanitarian-assistance-report-2023/

11. Maxwell J, Reuveny R. Resource scarcity and conflict in developing countries. J Peace Res. 2000;37(3):301–22. https://doi.org/10.1177/0022343300037003002.

12. Disasters Emergency Committee. Haiti, 3 years on. 2013 [accessed 14 July 2023]. Available from: https://www.dec.org.uk/story/haiti-3-years-on

13. UNESCO. Migrants, refugees, or displaced persons? 2021 [accessed 14 July 2023]. Available from: https://www.unesco.org/en/articles/migrants-refugees-or-displaced-persons

14. European Commission. Forced displacement: refugee, asylum-seekers and internally displaced people (IDPs). Belgium: European Civil Protection and Humanitarian Aid Operations; 2020. Available from: https://civil-protection-humanitarian-aid.ec.europa.eu/what/humanitarian-aid/ forced-displacement_en

15. The UN Refugee Agency. Global trends forced displacement in 2018. Geneva: Division of Programme Support and Management; 2019. Available from: https://www.unhcr.org/statistics/ unhcrstats/5d08d7ee7/unhcr-global-trends-2018.html

16. Our World in Data. Refugee population by country or territory of Asylum, 2021. 2021 [accessed 14 July 2023]. Available from: https://ourworldindata.org/grapher/ refugee-population-by-country-or-territory-of-asylum

17. Mosel I, Holloway K. Dignity and humanitarian action in displacement. England: Overseas Development Institute; 2019. Available from: https://odi.org/en/publications/ dignity-and-humanitarian-action-in-displacement/

18. Sphere Association. The Sphere handbook: humanitarian charter and minimum standards in humanitarian response, fourth edition. Switzerland: Practical Action Publishing; 2018. Available from: https://spherestandards.org/wp-content/uploads/Sphere-Handbook-2018-EN.pdf

19. Oxley M. 2018. Supporting community resilience in armed conflict and protracted violence – putting dignity back into humanitarian assistance. Available from: https://thesolutionsjournal. com/?p=9805

20. Blakemore E. Who are the Rohingya people? 2019 [accessed 13 November 2020]. Available from: https://www.nationalgeographic.com/culture/people/reference/rohingya-people/

Chapter 21
Healthcare for Refugees and Asylum Seekers

Tia Spelman

21.1 Introduction

There are 231,597 refugees in the UK as of November 2022, according to United Nations High Commissioner for Refugees (UNHCR) statistics, and 127,421 pending asylum seekers [1]. In the UK, refugees and asylum seekers are entitled to free NHS healthcare. However, they face many barriers accessing the system, some of which this chapter will cover [2]. Due to their experiences, previous country and migration journey, refugees have a variety of *physical, mental and social health needs* that may differ from the general population.

Seventy-two per cent of people seeking asylum in 2021 were from 10 countries: Iran, Iraq, Eritrea, Albania, Syria, Afghanistan, Sudan, Vietnam, El Salvador and Pakistan (see Fig. 21.1) [3]. The data includes main applicants and dependents (spouse, civil partner or child of the main applicant).

21.2 Definitions [4]

Asylum seekers may ask for housing or accommodation, for example a house, flat or hostel but cannot choose where in the country they reside. Monetary support is available, as asylum seekers are generally not allowed to work, and is currently £45 per person, per week, so about *£6.40 a day for food, sanitation and clothing* [5].

Once a claim is agreed and refugee status is granted, they can work; however, their support is stopped *28 days after the claim is accepted*. They must also move out of their accommodation, if they were given somewhere as an asylum seeker [6].

T. Spelman (✉)
School of Medicine, Cardiff University, Cardiff, UK
e-mail: spelmantk@cardiff.ac.uk

© The Author(s), under exclusive license to Springer Nature
Switzerland AG 2024
A. Fiander, G. Fry (eds.), *A Healthcare Students Introduction to Global Health*,
https://doi.org/10.1007/978-3-031-66563-9_21

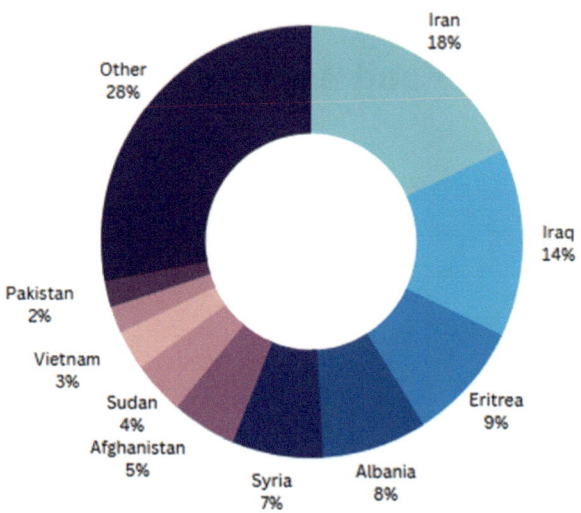

Iran 18%
Other 28%
Iraq 14%
Pakistan 2%
Vietnam 3%
Sudan 4%
Afghanistan 5%
Syria 7%
Albania 8%
Eritrea 9%

Definitions

Refugee	**Asylum seeker**	**Migrant**
A person who has fled their country due to serious violations of human rights or persecution. They have been granted **international protection**.	A person who has fled their country due to serious violations of human rights or persecution. They have **not yet been granted refugee status**, so in the UK they don't have the same rights as a British Citizen. Seeking asylum is a human right.	There is no universal correct definition of the word 'migrant'. It is often used as a term for someone who have moved from their country of origin, that aren't refugees or asylum seekers.

Fig. 21.1 Percentage of asylum claims from each country

21.3 What Barriers Do Refugees Face When Accessing Healthcare?

There are many barriers and difficulties that refugees face when accessing healthcare; these all impact the standard of healthcare and generally give rise to worsened health outcomes. The barriers will be grouped into the following categories or themes:

- Accessibility/affordability
- Language
- Stigma and discrimination
- Awareness of services

21.3.1   Accessibility/Affordability

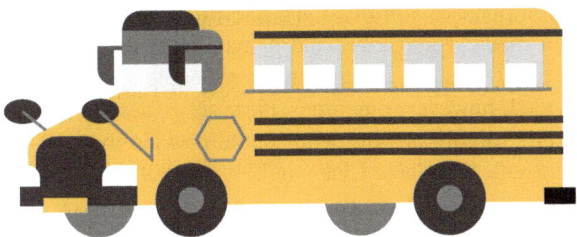

Although the health service is free for refugees and asylum seekers, asylum seekers often struggle to afford travel to and from the practice or hospital, due to the provision of £6.40 a day. If the practice is too far away, it means people cannot easily attend [7].

Then, if refugees can find a way to access the service, they must provide a HC2 letter which is a document that entitles them to free healthcare, but obtaining this is a lengthy process and an additional challenge if the patient does not speak English [7, 8].

In addition, accommodation that refugees are housed in were found to not meet basic standards, leading to worsened health, due to poor sanitation, inability to store medications and overcrowding. Mental health is also negatively impacted by these situations too: isolation and low standard of living contributing to this [9].

Ideally, refugees would be given a bigger budget to allow for situations such as these, thus improving ability to travel to health services. Housing quality should be assessed and improved; for example, ensure fewer people live in a shared space and ensure there are sufficient hygiene facilities for the number of refugees living there.

21.3.2   Language

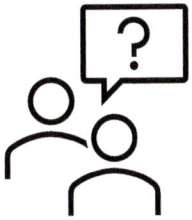

As reported in multiple studies, language barriers are significant. Although English Language classes (ESOL) are available, these may not be easy to access and the funding for the provision of these classes has dramatically decreased from £212.3m in 2008 to £105m in 2018 [10].

Even initially, obtaining an appointment and registering at a practice are challenging, and patients generally rely on family or friends who can speak English [11]. Using family and friends in place of a professional interpreter is not ideal, as they are not usually trained in medical language, and it may be difficult for the patient to open up about potentially sensitive issues in front of people they know.

Interpreters should be provided; however sometimes, there are issues coordinating them which can be attributed to not knowing who should provide them. If an interpreter is not physically present, Language Line can be used, but this in itself can be complicated and fail as technology does. Even with an interpreter, you rely on the accurate translation of medical terminology, and they may not be without bias [7, 11].

21.4   Awareness

As refugees come from various countries with different healthcare systems, they may be neither familiar with the structure of the NHS nor be aware that services are free for asylum seekers and refugees. This makes it difficult to navigate the service, and knowing where to go and how to get an appointment can be difficult [7].

In addition, with the various specialties and routes to a referral, they may not know which service is appropriate leading to unsuitable presentations at the Emergency Department. When charges are incorrectly applied, people may not understand how and when to complain, so may end up paying for a service that ought to be free.

Again, the language barrier can pose other problems; finding information can be made much harder as most of the information available is written in English.

21.5   Stigma and Discrimination

Stigma and Discrimination

The stigmatisation of accessing healthcare for refugees is a theme in many studies, particularly with mental health conditions [12]. Some refugees will also face discrimination due to race, accent or low proficiency of the host country's language, which can result in poorer care [13]. In one study, the participants felt staff were less sensitive to their conditions on account of racial discrimination [13].

Furthermore, staff often have insufficient knowledge of service provision for refugees as there is no formal training on the changing regulations. For example, a study in 2017 showed that although you don't have to declare immigration status to

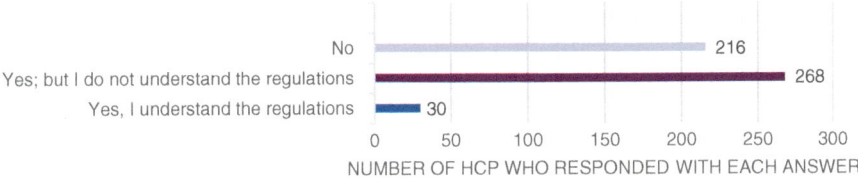

Fig. 21.2 Healthcare professional responses to survey regarding asylum seeker and refugee healthcare access [14]

register with a General Practice, 13% of migrants were refused registration because of their status [14] (Fig. 21.2).

In the same study, they asked healthcare professionals this question with the following response:

In summary, any refugee, asylum seeker, failed asylum seeker and their dependent(s), who receive support from the Home Office, are all exempt from NHS charges.

21.6   Healthcare Needs

On average, the health needs and common conditions of refugees and asylum seekers differ greatly from the general UK public and are usually more complex. This is due to a multitude of factors including their journeys to the UK, previous traumatic experiences, poor nutrition and hygiene due to poor funding and housing, poor management of chronic conditions and many more [15].

According to the World Health Organisation, the most common conditions seen in refugees include:

- Mental health conditions (post-traumatic stress disorder (PTSD), depression, anxiety)
- Communicable diseases (HIV, hepatitis B and C, tuberculosis, malaria)
- Chronic non-communicable diseases (diabetes, hypertension, dyslipidaemia)
- Women's health conditions such as Female Genital Mutilation (FGM) [16]

The prevalence of these conditions varies from country to country but is overall more prevalent in the refugee population. In one study, for instance, the incidence of tuberculosis in the migrant population in Alberta, Canada, was *four times higher* than the incidence in the host population [17].

21.6.1 Mental Health

It is estimated that 31% of displaced people have PTSD, 31% have depression, 11% have anxiety and 1.5% have psychosis [18]. Unfortunately, these seem to persist irrespective of how long ago they have been displaced (Fig. 21.3).

As seen in the graph, PTSD and depressive disorders are considerably more prevalent in refugees—understandably because of their often-difficult pasts, complicated by the transition into a new country, where perhaps they are isolated, or lack social support.

Some cultural differences make it more difficult for people to seek help, so care must be taken when having conversations about mental health. To ensure refugees get the help they need, healthcare professionals endeavour to remove unnecessary barriers. Healthcare professionals can do this by communicating calmly and sensitively and encourage the formation of a good rapport.

21.7 Health Outcomes: Sexual Health

There are many known differences in health outcomes for refugees, but this chapter will focus on specifically sexual health. Refugees often have more complex sexual and reproductive health needs, owing due causes such as lack of prior care, previous trauma and cultural sensitivities. Women who have been forcibly misplaced are much more likely to have experienced sexual and gender-based violence, which can lead to psychological problems, sexually transmitted infections (STIs) and trauma. Examples of this are FGM, rape, sexual assault and forced sex work [20].

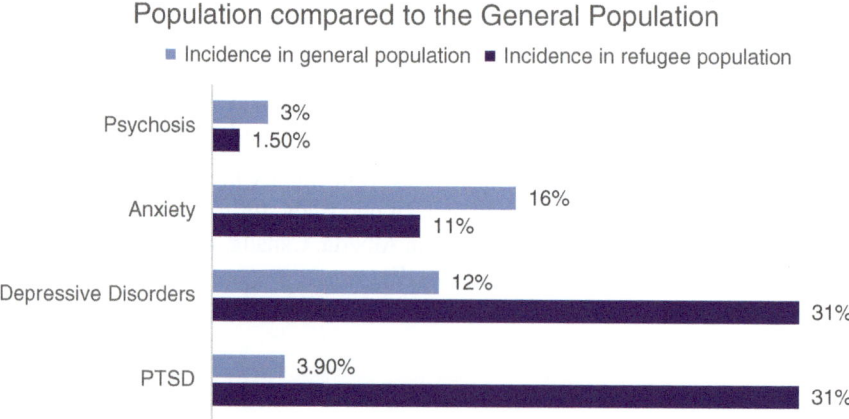

Fig. 21.3 Incidence of mental health conditions in refugee population compared to the general population [19]

According to the UK government website guidance [20], reasons refugees may not receive care are:

- Lack of awareness of services
- Re-traumatisation
- Fear of confidentiality breach
- Mistrust of healthcare professionals

The NHS offers different free sexual health services that people from other countries could not be aware of such as Frisky Wales (STI tests posted to an address), human papillomavirus (HPV) vaccinations for people under 18 and free contraception. Since COVID-19 pandemic, many places no longer offer walk-in services, so people must navigate the system and book an appointment.

21.7.1 An Example: Syphilis

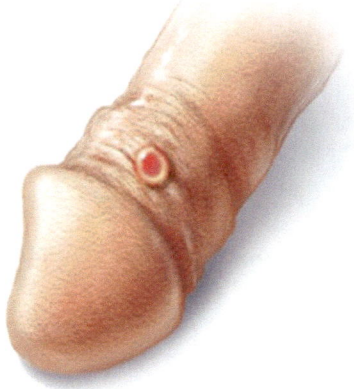

Image 1: chancre – Mayo Clinic [21]

Syphilis is an STI caused by the bacterium *Treponema pallidum*; it typically presents initially with a painless ulcer in the anogenital region called a *chancre* (see image [21]), but this can vary and is otherwise known as 'the great imitator' as it can generate a multitude of symptoms [22].

Secondary syphilis can lead to a widespread rash, and tertiary syphilis can cause neurological or cardiological problems too.

It is primarily spread through sexual contact, but also spread congenitally.

Refugees, in general, have a higher incidence of syphilis than the general population. In one study, it showed the incidence in pregnant refugees in a camp in Ethiopia was as high as 11.8% [23], compared to 1.11% in the general public [24]. This could be due to many reasons: lack of testing, lack of barrier contraception use, lack of treatment or just a general unawareness of safe sex practices. In pregnant people, it is important to avoid mother-to-child transmission. We can do this by increasing screening in refugee camps, and empowering people with information and the knowledge that they can get tested free of charge with a simple finger-prick test.

Specific services can be implemented for refugees or asylum seekers with longer appointments, translators readily available and doctors/healthcare professionals trained in refugee health, so they are aware of cultural sensitivities.

21.8   What Services and Guidance Are Already Available

There is a document provided by the Office for Health Improvement and Disparities to educate people about vulnerable migrant healthcare which provides links to various charities who specialise in this topic [25].

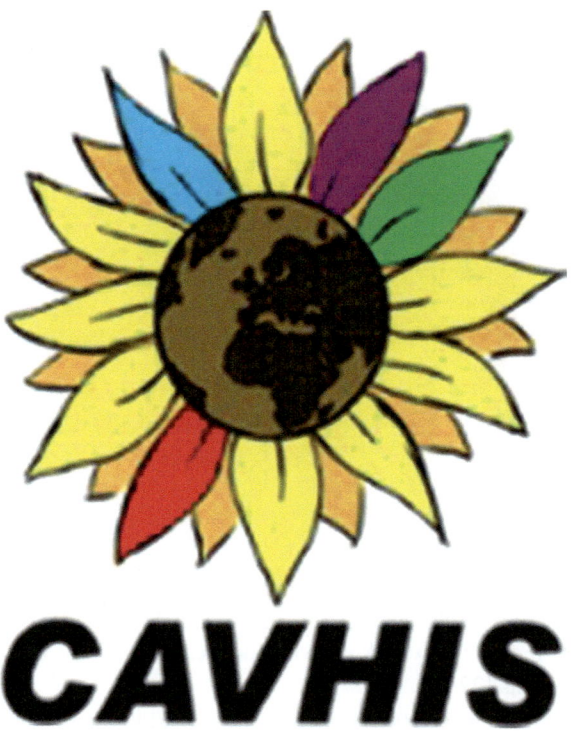

An example of refugee-based services is the *Cardiff and Vale Health Inclusion service (CAVHIS):* an organisation comprising of healthcare professionals who primarily provide screening for refugees and asylum seekers [26]. The initial appointment is with a senior nurse who takes a detailed history and initial investigations such as bloods, to screen for communicable diseases and so on.

The patient has the time and space to explore their health concerns with a translator, in their own language, and referrals can be made to relevant specialities and can register with a GP. There is also a midwife, who can deliver pregnancy care and screen for female genital mutilation.

There are several services like these throughout the country; this allows refugees to go to a specific place where the staff are experienced in this type of care and are informed of the laws regarding charges and usually non-discriminatory. They will also be more aware of cultural differences, therefore more sensitive to the needs of the patient, making them feel more comfortable and less judged.

21.9   What More Can We Do?

Medical Education

- Introduce mandatory training for refugee or asylum seeker healthcare into the medical education programme; this should **increase staff awareness** of the barriers into healthcare and improve knowledge of differing health needs of refugees.
- Encourage Equality and Diversity training, with regular updates. This should reduce bias from staff and make refugees feel more comfortable accessing NHS services.

More Services

- Increase number of Health Inclusion Services. Could potentially have GPs with sessions specifically for refugees, with increased appointment time to allow for more complex needs and translators readily available.
- Advertise the NHS Low Income scheme, which helps patients who can't afford transport get to appointments.

Raise Awareness

- Attend refugee community centres or sessions and encourage people to engage with healthcare, with leaflets and information printed in their language. For instance, in Cardiff, there is a student-led charity who gives talks to refugees about accessing healthcare so they feel more confident attending appointments.

References

1. Refugees UNHC for. Asylum in the UK [Internet]. UNHCR. [cited 2023 Feb 21]. Available from: https://www.unhcr.org/uk/asylum-in-the-uk.html
2. Refugees' and asylum seekers' entitlement to NHS care – Refugee and asylum seeker patient health toolkit – BMA [Internet]. The British Medical Association is the trade union and professional body for doctors in the UK. [cited 2023 Feb 21].

Available from: https://www.bma.org.uk/advice-and-support/ethics/refugees-overseas-visitors-and-vulnerable-migrants/refugee-and-asylum-seeker-patient-health-toolkit/refugees-and-asylum-seekers-entitlement-to-nhs-care

3. Asylum and refugee resettlement in the UK [Internet]. Migration Observatory. [cited 2023 Mar 21]. Available from: https://migrationobservatory.ox.ac.uk/resources/briefings/migration-to-the-uk-asylum/

4. Who is a refugee, a migrant or an asylum seeker? [Internet]. Amnesty International. [cited 2023 Feb 21]. Available from: https://www.amnesty.org/en/what-we-do/refugees-asylum-seekers-and-migrants/

5. Asylum support [Internet]. GOV.UK. [cited 2023 Feb 21]. Available from: https://www.gov.uk/asylum-support/what-youll-get

6. After you get refugee status [Internet]. Citizens Advice. [cited 2023 Mar 21]. Available from: https://www.citizensadvice.org.uk/immigration/after-you-get-refugee-status/

7. Kang C, Tomkow L, Farrington R. Access to primary health care for asylum seekers and refugees: a qualitative study of service user experiences in the UK. Br J Gen Pract. 2019;69(685):e537–45.

8. NHS Low Income Scheme (LIS) [Internet]. nhs.uk. 2020 [cited 2023 Feb 24]. Available from: https://www.nhs.uk/nhs-services/help-with-health-costs/nhs-low-income-scheme-lis/

9. Jones L, Phillimore J, Fu L, Hourani J, Lessard-Phillips L, Tatem B. "They just left me." Asylum seekers, health, and access to healthcare in initial and contingency accommodation. London: Doctors of the World UK; 2022.

10. Action R. New research shows refugees suffering from lack of English classes, despite strong public support for action by government [Internet]. Refugee Action. 2019 [cited 2023 Mar 21]. Available from: https://www.refugee-action.org.uk/new-research-shows-refugees-suffering-from-lack-of-english-classes-despite-strong-public-support-for-action-by-government/

11. Cheng IH, Drillich A, Schattner P. Refugee experiences of general practice in countries of resettlement: a literature review. Br J Gen Pract. 2015;65(632):e171–6.

12. DeSa S, Gebremeskel AT, Omonaiye O, Yaya S. Barriers and facilitators to access mental health services among refugee women in high-income countries: a systematic review. Syst Rev. 2022;11(1):62.

13. Mangrio E, Sjögren FK. Refugees' experiences of healthcare in the host country: a scoping review. BMC Health Serv Res. 2017;17(1):814.

14. Tomkow LJ, Kang CP, Farrington RL, Wiggans RE, Wilson RJ, Pushkar P, et al. Healthcare access for asylum seekers and refugees in England: a mixed methods study exploring service users' and health care professionals' awareness. Eur J Public Health. 2020;30(3):527–32.

15. Unique health challenges for refugees and asylum seekers - Refugee and asylum seeker patient health toolkit – BMA [Internet]. The British Medical Association is the trade union and professional body for doctors in the UK. [cited 2023 Mar 23]. Available from: https://www.bma.org.uk/advice-and-support/ethics/refugees-overseas-visitors-and-vulnerable-migrants/refugee-and-asylum-seeker-patient-health-toolkit/unique-health-challenges-for-refugees-and-asylum-seekers

16. Refugees UNHC for. Refugee health [Internet]. UNHCR. [cited 2023 Mar 23]. Available from: https://www.unhcr.org/excom/scaf/3ae68bf424/refugee-health.html

17. Asadi L, Heffernan C, Menzies D, Long R. Effectiveness of Canada's tuberculosis surveillance strategy in identifying immigrants at risk of developing and transmitting tuberculosis: a population-based retrospective cohort study. Lancet Public Health. 2017;2(10):e450–7.

18. Asylum seeker and refugee mental health | Royal College of Psychiatrists [Internet]. www.rcpsych.ac.uk. [cited 2023 Mar 23]. Available from: https://www.rcpsych.ac.uk/international/humanitarian-resources/asylum-seeker-and-refugee-mental-health

19. Blackmore R, Boyle JA, Fazel M, Ranasinha S, Gray KM, Fitzgerald G, et al. The prevalence of mental illness in refugees and asylum seekers: A systematic review and meta-analysis. PLoS Med. 2020;17(9):e1003337.

20. Women's health: migrant health guide [Internet]. GOV.UK. 2021 [cited 2023 Mar 15]. Available from: https://www.gov.uk/guidance/womens-health-migrant-health-guide

21. Syphilis – Symptoms and causes [Internet]. Mayo Clinic. [cited 2023 Mar 22]. Available from: https://www.mayoclinic.org/diseases-conditions/syphilis/symptoms-causes/syc-20351756

22. Syphilis infection – Symptoms, diagnosis and treatment I BMJ Best Practice [Internet]. [cited 2023 Mar 22]. Available from: https://bestpractice.bmj.com/topics/en-gb/50

23. Tadesse A, Geda A. Why Syphilis infection is high among pregnant women in refugee camps? A case in Ethiopia. Int J Womens Health. 2022;1(14):481–9.

24. Smolak A, Rowley J, Nagelkerke N, Kassebaum NJ, Chico RM, Korenromp EL, et al. Trends and predictors of Syphilis prevalence in the general population: global pooled analyses of 1103 prevalence measures including 136 million Syphilis tests. Clin Infect Dis Off Publ Infect Dis Soc Am. 2018;66(8):1184–91.

25. Vulnerable migrants: migrant health guide [Internet]. GOV.UK. [cited 2023 Mar 22]. Available from: https://www.gov.uk/guidance/vulnerable-migrants-migrant-health-guide

26. Service we provide [Internet]. Cardiff and Vale University Health Board. [cited 2023 Mar 22]. Available from: https://cavuhb.nhs.wales/our-services/cardiff-and-vale-health-inclusion-service/health-screening-for-asylum-seekers/service-we-provide/

Chapter 22
The Shortage of Healthcare Workers in Low Resource Countries

Lara Wiggins and Manaahil Sohail

22.1 Introduction

22.1.1 The Current Situation

- There is a critical shortage of healthcare workers in 57 countries, amounting to a global deficit of 2.4 million doctors, nurses and midwives.
- The areas most affected by these inequities are Sub-Saharan Africa and South-East Asia [1] (Figs. 22.1 and 22.2).

> **Case Study Example—Africa**
> - The number of healthcare workers in Africa is just 1,640,000 compared to 16,630,000 in Europe.
> - The ratio of nurses to doctors in Africa is 8:1.
> - In Sudan, in 2016, the number of medical doctors per 10,000 people was 2.63.
> - Africa has 24% of the burden of the disease, but only 3% of health workers and less than 1% of world expenditure.
> - Africa also has a severe level of disease—TB rates are high; malaria is endemic, and 72% of the AIDS deaths occur in Africa.
> - Extreme shortage of HCW—an estimated 720,000 physicians.
> - An increase of almost 140% is necessary to meet the threshold of healthcare workers needed [1].

L. Wiggins (✉) · M. Sohail
School of Medicine, Cardiff University, Cardiff, UK
e-mail: wigginsle@cardiff.ac.uk; sohailm1@cardiff.ac.uk

A. Fiander, G. Fry (eds.), *A Healthcare Students Introduction to Global Health*,
https://doi.org/10.1007/978-3-031-66563-9_22

219

**Figs. 22.1 and
22.2** Africa's burden of
the world's disease,
Africa's share of the
world's health
workforce [1]

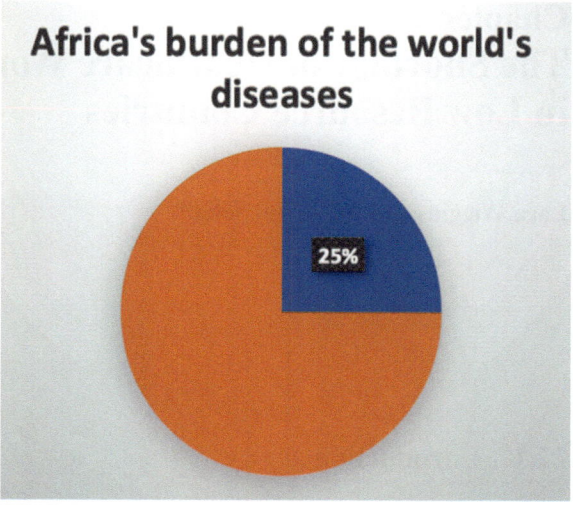

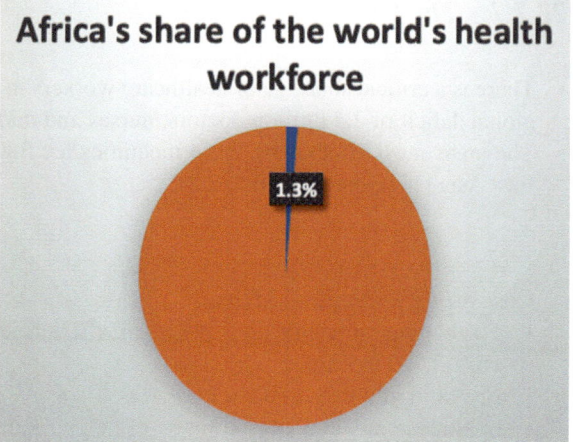

These graphs show that Africa has a large disease burden—25% of global disease, but only 1.3% of the global health workforce to manage such diseases. This is a large disparity contributing to poor health outcomes.

- Figure 22.3 shows that continents, such as Africa, have a significantly lower number of healthcare workers, health service providers and management/support workers compared with other continents such as Europe.
- For example, Europe has almost 11 times the number of healthcare providers compared to Africa and almost 16 times the number of healthcare workers.
- Figure 22.4 details the distribution of healthcare providers globally.
- Critical shortages are mostly seen in Sub-Saharan Africa and India.

WHO Region	Total Health Workforce Number	Total Health Workforce Density (per 1000)	Health Service Providers Number	Health Service Providers Percentage of total health workforce	Health Management and Support Workers Number	Health Management and Support Workers Percentage of total health workforce
Africa	1 640 000	2.3	1 360 000	83	280 000	17
Eastern Mediterranean	2 100 000	4.0	1 580 000	75	520 000	25
South-East Asia	7 040 000	4.3	4 730 000	67	2 300 000	33
Western Pacific	10 070 000	5.8	7 810 000	78	2 260 000	23
Europe	16 630 000	18.9	11 540 000	69	5 090 000	31
Americas	21 740 000	24.8	12 460 000	57	9 280 000	43
World	59 220 000	9.3	39 470 000	67	19 750 000	33

Fig. 22.3 Global health workforce by density [1]

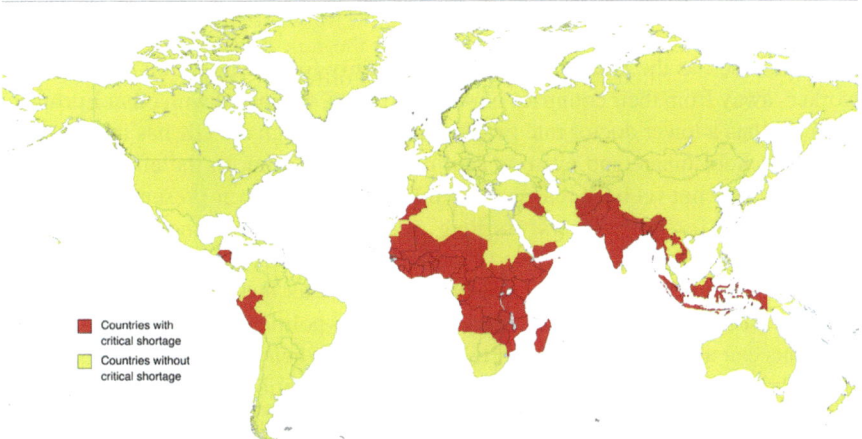

Fig. 22.4 Countries with a critical shortage of health service providers [1]

- Clear global disparities of healthcare worker coverage can be seen in Fig. 22.4. Large areas including many LRCs have critical shortages of healthcare workers, whereas the majority of the 'Western World' has no critical shortages.

As you can see from Fig. 22.4, there is an unequal distribution of healthcare workers across the world.

- Rural/Urban divide: 85% of doctors and 65% of nurses are in urban areas.
- Fifty-seven countries are below a threshold of meeting 80% healthcare coverage level—translating to a critical shortage.
- To meet 100% coverage, these countries would need a global increase of 4.3 million health workers.
- The greatest shortages can be seen in SE Asia (Bangladesh, India and Indonesia), and the largest relative need occurs in Sub-Saharan Africa [1].

The financial situation and spending on Health

- Highest health spending: North America, Western Europe and Oceania.
- Lowest health spending: West, Central and East Africa, and South Asia.
- The cost of training healthcare workers however is often higher in LRCs.
- For example, the average cost of training healthcare workers per year per country is 136 million US dollars. However, in countries such as India, the cost incurred is 2 billion US dollars per year [1].

22.2 Reasons for the Shortage of Healthcare Workers

22.2.1 Migration

Countries such as the UK hold some responsibility for the migration of healthcare workers away from their countries of origin. The UK compared with other European countries has a lower doctor rate per population. Although the UK has increased its medical school intake and even created new medical schools, the effects of these strategies have not yet been realised. Therefore, there is an ever-present demand and 'poaching' of foreign workers. As long as shortages exist in the UK, there will always be a pull factor for workers to migrate and work in the UK [2].

Pull factors include higher standards of living, better quality of life, higher salaries and access to advanced technology. The socio-political and professional environments can also be more stable. Push factors from their country of origin include higher levels of stress, greater workload and low motivation due to a comparatively poor salary. The subsequent 'brain drain'—that is loss of well-educated working professionals—affects the standard of education in the country for the next generation.

This also contributes to what academics describe as 'a medical carousel' [3]. This term describes the following: a doctor from an urban setting migrates to a country with higher standards of living. A doctor from a rural setting within the same country fills the vacancy. This leaves the least desirable position in the rural area vacant.

22.2.2 Education

Replacing these doctors has been made difficult by the expansion of private medical schools in low- and middle-income countries. Access to higher education is impossible for students from low economic backgrounds, and therefore, the opportunity of a career in healthcare is open to only the wealthy.

22.2.3 Presence of Unqualified Healthcare Workers or Traditional Healers

In LRCs, people often turn to traditional remedies or faith healers rather than seeking professional medical help. This is often seen in the case of mental health treatment. Therefore, this reduces the demand for professional healthcare workers in this setting.

India Case Study [4]

A hospital-based study in Gwalior, India, enrolled 295 patients suffering from severe mental illnesses and identified significant barriers to them seeking medical care. The first barrier to seeking care was the distance to mental health services. The mean distance travelled by the patients was 249 km, indicating restricted access to mental health treatments in India. For many of these patients, psychiatric care was not their first point of care. Approximately 68.5% of the patients in the study consulted faith healers before attending the hospital. The low socioeconomic backgrounds and illiteracy of many of the patients contributed to their reluctance to seek treatment.

It has been found that in India, many traditional healers do not admit their inability to treat mental illness. They mislead patients and their families by claiming that these illnesses have supernatural causes and not medical issues. This in turn depletes the demand for professional healthcare workers in these settings.

22.3 Solutions for the Shortage of Healthcare Providers (HCPs)

1. Influence of the Western world

Western countries such as the UK must recognise their contribution to the 'brain drain' from low resource countries. The first solution is to further increase medical, nursing and midwifery school capacity in the UK, therefore reducing UK dependence on overseas recruitment of healthcare workers.

UK universities and hospitals have begun to create mutually beneficial links between themselves and institutions in Africa to make healthcare an attractive prospective career for future generations of HCPs in LRC. Strategies such as these require the support of the World Health Organisation and other high-income countries in tackling the push/pull factors from LRCs.

2. Bonding system

A bonding system necessitates that HCPs serve in the country of training for a certain period of time before they leave to study or work elsewhere. This means that their country of origin reaps some benefit from investing in the individual's training. This scheme also increases the likelihood of the doctors staying long term.

3. Incentives

Governments may offer incentives to encourage healthcare workers to stay in their country of origin. Some of the potential incentives include:

- Travel from rural areas to cities
- Provision of accommodation
- Better wages
- Scholarships
- Educating members of society to encourage and support health workers and patients .

Case Study
In the Philippines, the government set up The Philippine Overseas Employment Administration which obligated professionals working abroad to send back remittances. In 2004, these remittances accounted for up to 10% of Gross Domestic Product per capita (GDP), and they were re-invested in the country's own infrastructure. The scheme was accompanied by privileges such as loans at preferential rates and tax-free shopping. Collectively, this encouraged skilled migrants to return and work for the Philippine healthcare system.

4. Education and Training: The Introduction of Mid-Level Workers (MLWs)

- MLWs are present globally as Physician Assistants in America; Clinical Officers in Africa; Lady Health Workers in Pakistan and Tecnicos de Cirugia providing surgical care in Mozambique. They are certified individuals who are not doctors but have been trained to diagnose and manage common health problems, manage emergency care or refer the patient as necessary.
- Both unskilled and skilled workers can train to be a clinical officer, with average training for an unskilled worker being 2–4 years.
- Over 10,000 Clinical Officers have been trained in Uganda, Tanzania and Kenya. In many LRCs, they have been shown to be an integral part of the healthcare system, greatly improving access to care.
- MLWs can improve healthcare coverage and work within a doctor led team. As they do not hold a transferable qualification, they are unable to migrate as easily, and studies have shown they are more likely to remain than doctors.
- One example of where MLWs were successful was in the HIV crisis in Africa [5].

5. Collaboration Between Organisations and Governments

The Working for Health Programme 2017–2021

This is an example of collaboration between organisations as a joint WHO, International Labour Organisation (ILO) and Organization for Economic Cooperation and Development (OECD) programme with the vision to 'Accelerate progress towards universal health coverage and attaining the goals of the 2030 Agenda for Sustainable Development by ensuring equitable access to health workers within strengthened health systems' using a 5-year action plan from 2017 to 2021 [6]. The organisations sought to engage in technical cooperation, capacity development, research, facilitation of investments and financing and normative guidance for member states.

WHO—Working Together for Health

In 2006, the WHO set out a 10-year action plan for governments entitled: 'Working Together for Health' as set out below. The decade goal for all countries was to build high-performing workforces for national health systems to respond to current and emerging challenges. The action plan highlights the need for coordination between countries and global solidarity to improve the healthcare worker shortage in LRCs (Fig. 22.5).

6. Financial Solutions

In the working Together for Health Action plan, the WHO notes: 'The magnitude of the health workforce crisis in the world's poorest countries cannot be overstated and requires an urgent, sustained and coordinated response from the international community. Donors must facilitate immediate and longer-term financing of human resources as a health systems investment. A 50:50 guideline is recommended, whereby 50% of all international assistance funds are devoted to health systems, with half of this funding devoted to national health workforce strengthening strategies' [1].

		2006 Immediate	2010 Mid-Point	2015 Decade
Country leadership	Management	Cut waste, improve incentives	Use effective management practices	Sustain high performance workforce
	Education	Revitalise education stratgies	Strengthen accreditation and licensing	Prepare workforce for the future
	Planning	Design national workforce strategies	Overcome barriers to implementation	Evaluate and redesign strategies, based on robust national capacity
Global solidarity	Knowledge and learning	Develop common technical frameworks	Asess performance with comparable metrics	Share evidence based good practises
		Pool Expertise	Fund priority research	Share evidence based good practises
	Enabling policies	Advocate ethical recruitment and migrant workers rights	Adhere to responsible recruitment guidelines	Manage increased migratory flows for equity and fairness
		Pursue final sapce exceptionality	Expand fiscal space for health	Support fiscal sustainability
	Crisis response	Finance national plans fir 25% if crisis counties	Expand financing to half of crisis countries	Support financing for national plans of all countries in crisis
		Agree on best donor resource practices for human resources for health	Adopt 50-50 investment guideline for priority programmes	Support financing for national plans of all countries in crisis

Fig. 22.5 The ten-year plan of action [1]

7. Retaining Healthcare Workers in LRC

The WHO discusses the labour market for human resources for health in low-
and middle-income countries and gives examples of how some countries have gone
about retaining healthcare workers [7].

Thailand Case Study
- Initial shortage of workers due to lack of compensation, higher salaries and more
  prestigious jobs in other professions
- Thailand's Ministry of Health—reallocated federal funds towards training and
  retaining of health workers

Kenya Case Study
- Unfilled rural posts; Kenyan government did not have the funds to increase train-
  ing and employment in these areas.
- The Ministry of Health used external donor resources to initiate an Emergency
  Hiring Programme.
- Secure 3-year contract for healthcare workers to work in understaffed rural
  regions. Applicants interviewed in home regions rather than travel to the capital
  Nairobi.
- Ministry of Health implemented hardship allowances for rural areas, housing
  grants and two sessions of paid leave.
- This scheme aims to offset wage deficits between rural and urban areas.

Rwanda Case Study
- An issue in Rwanda was the presence of 'ghost workers' who received funding
  from the government via salaries, but which had little impact on quality of care
  due to absenteeism.
- Pay-for-performance strategies were implemented in Rwanda and other countries to eradicate these workers and replace them with workers who are paid for
  the time they work in public clinics.
- This has led to a dramatic reduction in ghost workers and improvements in quan-
  tity and quality of care.

8. An Increased Focus on Primary Care and Community-Based Initiatives

One strategy to improve access is an increased focus on primary care and
community-based initiatives. An example of this is the implementation of
Community Health Worker (CHW) programmes [5]. Community-based health
workers (CHWs) are referred to by a variety of names, such as health auxiliaries,
health volunteers, health promoters, family welfare educators, village health workers and community lay health aides. They are involved in providing preventive medical services, monitoring the community's health, identifying patients at particular

risk and providing basic treatment services. It is important that CHWs work as part of a primary care team and that their work is recognized, supervised and rewarded.

- CHW programmes were effective in Malaria testing in Zambia, 2006, which enabled fast detection and avoided overtreatment.
- There is good evidence that CHWs can undertake various tasks contributing to child survival. Examples include management of childhood illness and delivery of preventive interventions such as immunisation.
- A study in Western Cape Province, South Africa, showed that CHW teams are cost effective, especially with infectious disease such as TB [5].

22.4   The Future of the Healthcare Shortage in LRCs

Health systems can only function with health workers; improving health service coverage and realizing the right to the enjoyment of the highest attainable standard of health are dependent on their availability, accessibility, acceptability and quality [8].

22.4.1   The United Nation's Sustainable Development Goals (SDGs) Implementation and Progress

One of the UN's SDGs (Goal 3c) was to 'Increase health financing and support health workforce in developing countries'. The UN has provided maps to track the progress of this goal, comparing the healthcare provider density in 2000 to that in 2019 (Figs. 22.6 and 22.7) (Goal 3: Good Health and Well-Being - SDG Tracker. 2021).

- From these maps, it can be seen that there is an HCP divide, with Europe having a high density of healthcare coverage (ranging from 4 to 6 doctors per 1000 people) compared with Asia and Africa, and parts of South America (ranging from 0 to 3 doctors per 1000 people). High resource countries such as Sweden have some of the highest densities of doctors (4.89 per 1000).
- Libya has seen an increase in HCPs, from 1.24 medical doctors per 1000 in 2000 to 2.09 per 1000 in 2016.
- There is absent data in 2016 compared to 2000 for some countries, in Africa especially, making it hard to determine improvement in HCPs.

- (Goal 3: Good Health and Well-Being - SDG Tracker, 2021)

Medical doctors per 1,000 people, 2000

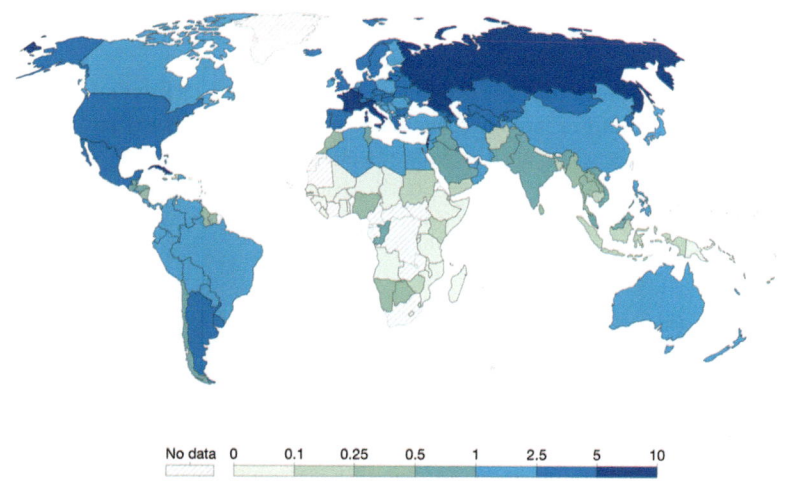

Source: Data compiled from multiple sources by World Bank   OurWorldInData.org/financing-healthcare · CC BY
Note: Medical doctors include generalist physicians and specialist medical practitioners.

Fig. 22.6 Medical doctors per 1000 people, *2000* (Goal 3: Good Health and Well-Being – SDG Tracker)

Medical doctors per 1,000 people, 2019

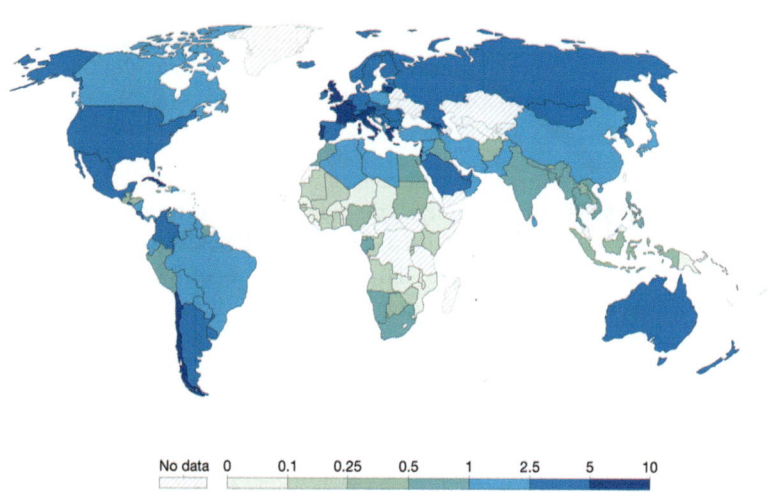

Source: Data compiled from multiple sources by World Bank   OurWorldInData.org/financing-healthcare · CC BY
Note: Medical doctors include generalist physicians and specialist medical practitioners.

Fig. 22.7 Medical doctors per 1000 people, *2019* (Goal 3: Good Health and Well-Being – SDG Tracker)

22.4.2 The WHO Global Strategy on Human Resources for Health: Workforce 2030

The WHO has put in place a strategy that should accelerate progress towards universal health coverage and relevant UN SDGs by 2030. Its vision is to ensure equitable access to health workers within strengthened health systems. It recognises that the health workforce has a vital role in building the resilience of communities and health systems to respond to disasters caused by natural or man-made hazards, as well as related environmental, technological and biological hazards and risks. Despite progress, there is still a need to boost political will and mobilize resources for the health workforce, including the planning, education, management and reward of HCPs. The vision that by 2030 all communities have universal access to health workers, without stigma and discrimination, requires combining the adoption of effective policies at national, regional and global levels with adequate investment to address unmet needs.

References

1. World Health Organisation. The world health report : 2006: working together for health. Geneva, Switzerland: WHO Document Production Services; 2006. Available from: https://www.who.int/publications-detail-redirect/9241563176
2. Witt J. Addressing the migration of health professionals: the role of working conditions and educational placements. BMC Public Health. 2009;9 Suppl 1(Suppl 1):S7. https://doi.org/10.1186/1471-2458-9-S1-S7. PMID: 19922691; PMCID: PMC2779509
3. Eastwood JB, Conroy RE, Naicker S, West PA, Tutt RC, Plange-Rhule J. Loss of health professionals from sub-Saharan Africa: the pivotal role of the UK. Lancet. 2005;365(9474):1893–900. https://doi.org/10.1016/S0140-6736(05)66623-8.
4. Lahariya C, Singhal S, Gupta S, Mishra A. Pathway of care among psychiatric patients attending a mental health institution in central India. Indian J Psychiatry. 2010;52(4):333–8. https://doi.org/10.4103/0019-5545.74308. PMID: 21267367; PMCID: PMC3025159
5. Bangdiwala SI, Fonn S, Okoye O, Tollman S. Workforce resources for health in developing countries. Public Health Rev. 2010;32:296–318. https://doi.org/10.1007/BF03391604.
6. World Health Organization, 2018. Five-year action plan for health employment and inclusive economic growth (2017–2021). Available at: https://www.who.int/publications/i/item/9789241514149
7. World Health Organisation, 2012. The Labour market for human resources in low- and middle-income countries. Human Resources for Health Observer 11. Geneva, Switzerland: WHO Document Production Services. Available at: https://cdn.who.int/media/docs/default-source/health-workforce/2012-hrh-journal-labour-market.pdf?sfvrsn=68a057af_1&download=true
8. World Health Organisation 2016. The Global strategy on human resources for health: workforce 2030. Geneva, Switzerland: WHO Document Production Services. Available at: https://www.who.int/publications/i/item/9789241511131

Chapter 23
Aid: A Blessing, or a Curse?

Tashlyn De Almeida Pereira and Lydia Benitez-Jones

23.1 An Introduction to Aid

23.1.1 What Is Aid?

The term 'aid' is known as economic help that more resourced countries supply to less resourced countries. This chart (Fig. 23.1) with data from the OECD (Organisation for Economic Co-operation and development) shows governmental aid broken down. Economic development takes up the largest area by far. However, the different sections of this chart are not independent from one another; they are all interconnected and feed into each other with economic development being the key starting point for the other aspects to thrive. However, when this idea is put into practice, the situation is complex.

23.1.1.1 What Difference Does Aid Make?

Over US$1 trillion in development-related aid has been transferred in the past 50 years from more resourced countries to Africa. But has this made any substantial difference over this time? Unfortunately, not. Africans are poorer, and the economic rate of growth is slower. Many African countries are at least as poor as they were 40 years ago, with a per capita income average of around US$1 a day which is lower than their per capita income in the 1970s [2, 3].

Poverty greatly hinders progress towards the SDGs (Sustainable Development Goals) of the UN (United Nations). For example:

T. De Almeida Pereira (✉) · L. Benitez-Jones
School of Medicine, Cardiff University, Cardiff, UK
e-mail: tashlyn.dealmeidapereira3@wales.nhs.uk; Benitez-JonesL@cardiff.ac.uk

© The Author(s), under exclusive license to Springer Nature   231
Switzerland AG 2024
A. Fiander, G. Fry (eds.), *A Healthcare Students Introduction to Global Health*,
https://doi.org/10.1007/978-3-031-66563-9_23

Chart showing governmental aid broken down by type (in %)

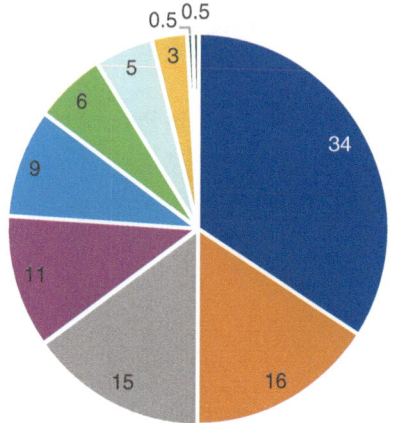

- Economic development
- Health
- Humanitarian response and preparation
- Government and civil society
- Education
- Water and Sanitation
- Environment
- Conflict and Security
- Food aid
- Budget Support

Fig. 23.1 Pie chart showing the way that government aid is generally given from more resourced countries to less resource countries, and the way it is broken down throughout the world. Economic development is the most dominant sector of aid given by the government. Debt relief is not shown on this chart as it makes up close to 0% of governmental aid [1]

- Adult literacy has dropped across Africa below 1980s' levels.
- One in every 7 children dies under the age of 5 across the African continent.
- Africa is the only continent with a life expectancy lower than 60 years. However, this may be due to the devastating impact of the HIV-AIDS pandemic [2].

Before exploring the topic in more depth, let us look at the different types of aid that can be provided in the next section.

23.1.2   Types of Aid [2]

Aid can be classified into three main types:

- *Emergency or humanitarian aid*—It is given as a response and a means to assist after sudden disasters and catastrophes. For example, following the 2004 Asian tsunami.
- *Charity based aid*—When charitable organisations provide money to people or institutions. For example, OXFAM.
- *Systematic aid*—Aid payments are made to governments directly either through institutions such as the World Bank (termed as multilateral aid) or via transfers from governments to governments (known as bilateral aid).

In this pie chart (Fig. 23.2) seen below, bilateral aid is represented as the largest type of systematic aid with 58% in comparison to multilateral aid.

Fig. 23.2 Data from 2015 showing the way that systematic aid is broken down into and the proportion of each type of systematic aid generally throughout the world [1]

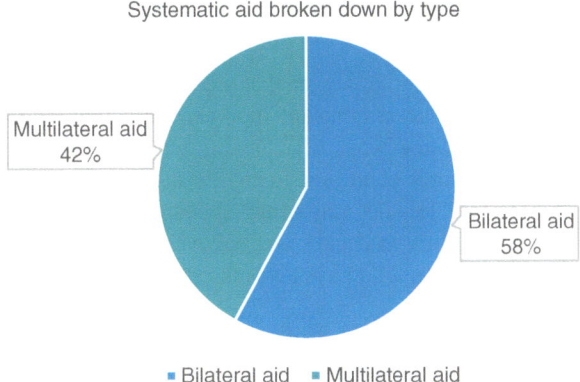

Systematic aid broken down by type

Although there are clear benefits to charity, this also attracts criticism. Charities are often criticised for elevated administrative costs, poor implementation and, on some occasions, for coercion to do their donor government's requests. For example, in 2005, the USA guaranteed US$15 billion over 5 years to combat AIDS. However, this help was conditional. Two-thirds of the money provided had to go to pro-abstinence programmes and would not be accessible to any organizations with clinics offering abortion services [2].

Furthermore, the money provided to African countries coming from emergency and charity aid is a small amount compared to the billions dispensed per year directly to the recipient countries' governments. This money transferred to African governments from wealthier countries is done in the form of grants (money given for nothing in return) or loans (which is often lent for longer periods than regular markets, and at lower interest rates).

23.1.2.1 Loans vs. Grants [2]

It is argued that loans encourage governments to wisely mobilise the money given, modify taxes and maintain the levels of revenue collection. This is in contrast to grants, which are viewed as free funds and therefore could substitute a government's domestic revenue [4].

It makes sense to think that poor countries' investments need a long maturation period before they begin to have the desired effect on the gross domestic product (GDP) to service loans. In fact, it has been argued by many scholars that it is due to the many loans, and not grants, received by African countries which has made them so heavily indebted and prevented them from achieving their development aims.

23.1.3 Does Aid Perpetuate Dependency?

There is, however, a danger that aid could lead to inactivity from policymakers. If aid is viewed as a constant income, policymakers may have less imperative in searching for new ways of achieving long-term development for their countries. In this case, poorer countries, being aid-dependent, have no need to pursue tax revenues. At first, less tax may sound appealing; however, in reality, the lack of taxation leads to a failure in checks and balances between the people and the governments. That is, a person who pays taxes is more likely to demand that their money gets put to good use.

This widespread aid-dependency culture encourages receiving countries to support unproductive public sectors as a way of pleasing the donor countries. There is a danger that this could amount to African countries being run indirectly by Western politicians rather than by themselves, for themselves.

23.2 Analysing Systematic Approaches to Aid

There have been countless different aid strategies deployed by governments and organisations, so it is crucial to examine some of the most successful strategies and identify effective and ineffective components. This allows us to gain a better understanding of what effective aid may look like.

23.2.1 Governmental Support—The International Development Association (IDA)

The IDA is an arm of the World Bank which supplies loans to poverty-stricken countries at a concessional interest rate. As of July 2020, there have been 37 graduates of this governmental programme. This means that these countries' financial status has improved enough that they no longer require any monetary aid from the IDA [5].

They categorise countries into three groups: those with high risk of debt distress (where a country's government is unable to repay their debt) will receive a full grant, those with medium risk of debt distress will receive a mixture between grants and loans, and those with low risk will receive a full loan.

Botswana

Of the 37 IDA graduate countries, Botswana is perhaps the most recognised success, having shown a Gross National Income (GNI) per capita increase from US$100 in 1967 to US$7020 in 2013 [6]. Botswana government used this aid to improve their trade policies, meaning that there was an increase in competition for both domestic and foreign investments (Table 23.1).

23.2.1.1 Governmental Support—Implementing Conditionalities

There have been strategies that do attempt to implement conditionalities (terms) in order to reduce corruption, but not with much success. For example, there was the Marshall plan (1948) and the international monetary fund (present).

Example: The Marshall Plan [7]
The Marshall plan was where America donated a large sum of grants to Germany and France so that they could rebuild their economy and infrastructure after the Second World War. However, there were a set of conditions that the recipient countries had to follow in order to receive this aid:

1. The recipient countries must spend the money from aid on specific goods that originate from the donor country.
2. The donor country can at any point choose/change the project in which aid will be given.
3. The recipient country must follow economic policies set out by the donor country.

Disadvantages of Conditionalities—Colonialism
Although it may prove successful, as in the cases of Germany and France, these systems may perpetuate the issue of *colonialism*. Colonialism refers to 'the practice by which a powerful country directly controls less powerful countries and uses their resources to increase its own power and wealth' [8]. The government may benefit

Table 23.1 Benefits and disadvantages of monetary aid from IDA [2]

Benefits	Disadvantages
Concessional interest rates By providing close to 0% interest rates, it allows countries to only repay what they have borrowed. This helps reduce the debt some countries may be in and reduces the potential for future debt distress.	*External factors influence the success of the grants/loans* Factors such as governmental corruption can influence how the country uses the money. They may not use the money for investments as Botswana did, and so the extra cash flow cannot guarantee that all governments would deploy the same strategy.
Debt sustainability Due to the categorisation process of the countries, it allows countries to receive funding irrespective of their debt status. This allows countries that may not normally be able to take loans out at such low interest rates to do so.	

from the monetary gain, but it has been argued that the local tradespeople who produce the goods for the country may be put out of business.

23.2.2 Healthcare Systems Support—Sector-Wide Approaches (SWAps)

An alternative to governmental–governmental aid, but still maintaining the systematic approach, is directly supporting the healthcare systems of LRCs through *sector-wide approaches (SWAps)*. This strategy targets universal health coverage (which is one of the targets set out by SDGs) by empowering LRCs' healthcare systems.

This is where donor countries and recipient countries pool money together to fund the health sector. Some countries that implemented this strategy are Zambia, Ghana and Bangladesh. The World Bank and World Health Organisation (WHO) consider this an integral part in providing effective aid for the healthcare sector in LRCs [9] (Table 23.2).

23.2.2.1 Healthcare Systems Support—Global Health Partnerships (GHP)

As well as bilateral donations from governments, there are partnerships between private organisations, LRC representatives and communities, which target-specific diseases by providing monetary aid. The purpose of creating an initiative such as these was to attract private investments and funding into global health. Examples of this are *Roll Back Malaria, the Vaccine Alliance* and *the Global Fund* [10, 11].

Table 23.2 Benefits and disadvantages of healthcare support from SWAPs

Benefits	Disadvantages
Governments are able to allocate funds to areas that need aid the most: The LRC governments may know where more resources need to be allocated within their own country.	*Negotiations between governments may fail:* This may lead to tension between donor and recipient countries.
Alleviation on the healthcare sector: The healthcare sector receives extra money; therefore, the pressure to allocate resources on a low budget is lessened.	*Resources allocated unfairly:* Money may be put into areas of the healthcare sector that are less productive, or overlook areas which may need to be better supported.
Governments supported with leadership and management: The LRC governments can then continue good leadership beyond the programme.	*Civilians and healthcare workers excluded from allocation of resources:* Civilians and healthcare workers will usually know most about what needs to improve within the system, so it may be unfair to exclude this input.

They Have Also Played a Role in Anti-Corruption

- If there is any corruption, or diversion of funds suspected, then they will distance themselves from the governments but continue to supply credits and funding to the representatives they are allied with.
- Healthcare in many LRCS has been highly underfunded in the past. But as some of the grants and credits are implemented with the help of communities, healthcare has been a higher priority in countries where GHPs are in place.

Promoting Sustainability and Resilience Through Aid

Perhaps, the best way to implement aid is by cutting out the middleman, the government. This is what this chapter will now explore.

23.2.3 Microfinancing

Microfinancing allows entrepreneurs in impoverished areas, who may not normally have access to traditional loan services, to take out small loans (known as microcredits). This allows for greater financial inclusion and greater opportunities for those with a lower income.

1. Provides entrepreneurs and small businesses with capital to expand their business.
2. Allows lower income individuals invest in themselves and build themselves up.

As money is being given directly to the individual rather than passing through the government and potentially corrupt policies, microfinancing empowers people to create themselves an income, consequently allowing them to provide for themselves and their families, and also invest in their countries' economy [12].

However, as with most aid schemes, there have been flaws.

- The microfinance industry has served only a small population of people.
- The interest rates on the loans tend to be higher than average bank loan rates.
- They are short term loans and often require quick repayments.

These drawbacks make microloans less appealing and have hindered its success thus far, because long-term investments (such as education) do not provide fast enough cash return. It means that recipients are not able to repay their loans in time.

23.2.3.1 Direct Giving (GiveDirectly) [13]

GiveDirectly is the world's first non-profit that allows donors to send their money directly to the people living in LRCs. They determine who to send money to by identifying the poorest villages and then enrolling all the households into the programme.

By using this method of charitable aid, the money ends up straight in the hands of the people rather than having to bypass potentially corrupt governments.

What Impact has This Form of Aid Had? (Fig. 23.3)

1. Sustainable Cash—as many of the recipients use the grants to invest in education, nutrition and small businesses, they are able to receive a steady income. They can then continue to use this income for other necessities to better themselves and their quality of life.
2. Reducing Aid Dependence—the production of an income is crucial in preventing aid dependence. Those with a stable income are less likely to have to rely on aid again and are more resilient.

As there are no conditions, there is no guarantee that the recipients will use this money for investments. Also, as governments are not involved, there are less large-scale community projects such as wells, sanitation building and healthcare investments.

What Is Effective Aid?

Perhaps, the answer to effective aid lies with direct cash transfers since this allows money to be given directly to those in true need, the people. Without involving governments and their allied organisations, sustainable aid may be achieved; people in LRCs can use the grants to give themselves stable incomes and support their own and their families' futures. This can allow stronger economic building and perhaps even a way out of poverty for many people, therefore reducing the likelihood of aid dependency in LRCs. As a direct result of this, the SDG of eradicating poverty by 2030 may be in reach [15].

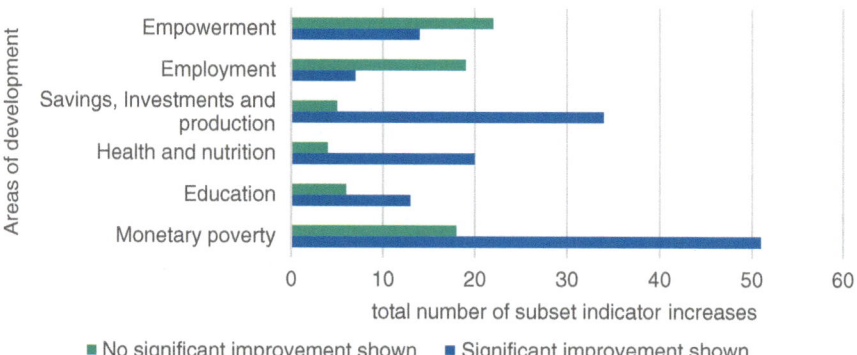

Fig. 23.3 Effects of cash transfers on different areas of development (Adapted from Overseas Development institute report 2016) [14]

Overall, effective aid is not a one-shoe-fits-all situation as different LRCs have different political, economic and environmental factors, and therefore, it would be unfair to rule out any method of giving aid. But by adopting and implementing direct giving as a more widely available option, we may start to see improvements.

References

1. Australian Council For International Development. Understanding Aid: Explanatory paper on international and Australian aid Australia 2017 [Available from: https://acfid.asn.au/sites/site.acfid/files/resource_document/ACFID%20Understanding%20Aid.pdf
2. Moyo D. Dead aid : why aid makes things worse and how there is another way for Africa. London: Penguin; 2010.
3. Lancaster C. Aid effectiveness in Africa: the unfinished agenda. J Afr Econ. 1999;8(4):487–503.
4. Clements B, Gupta S, Pivovarsky A, Tiongson ER. Foreign aid: grants versus loan. Finance and Development [Internet]. 2004.
5. International Development Association. IDA graduates 2021 [updated 20th March 2023. Available from: https://ida.worldbank.org/en/about/borrowing-countries/ida-graduates
6. The World Bank. Databank- World development Indicators. 2023.
7. Llewellyn J, Thompson S. The Marshall plan: Alpha history; 2020. Available from: https://alphahistory.com/coldwar/marshall-plan/
8. Collins Dictionary. 2023. Colonialism.
9. Peters DH, Paina L, Schleimann F. Sector-wide approaches (SWAps) in health: what have we learned? Health Policy Plan. 2013;28(8):884–90.
10. World Health Organization. Global Health Partnerships Europe.
11. Plamondon KM, Brisbois B, Dubent L, Larson CP. Assessing how global health partnerships function: an equity-informed critical interpretive synthesis. Global Health. 2021;17(1):73.
12. Campbell G. Microfinancing the developing world: how small loans empower local economies and catalyse neoliberalism's endgame. Third World Quart. 2010;31(7):1081–90.
13. GiveDirectly. Research on cash transfers: GiveDirectly; 2020 [updated 22nd December 2020. Available from: https://www.givedirectly.org/research-on-cash-transfers/
14. Bastagli F, Hagen-Zanker J, Harman L, Barca V, Sturge G, Schmidt T, et al. Cash transfers: what does the evidence say London: Overseas Development Institute (ODI); 2016. Available from: https://odi.org/en/publications/cash-transfers-what-does-the-evidence-say-a-rigorous-review-of-impacts-and-the-role-of-design-and-implementation-features/
15. High Level panel on Humanitarin cash transfers. Doing cash differently: how cash transfers can transform humanitarian aid: Overseas Development Institute (ODI); 2015. Available from: https://cdn.odi.org/media/documents/9828.pdf

Chapter 24
The Climate Crisis Is a Health Crisis

Umraj Rai and Natalie Olsen

Human activities have exploited the earth's resources at an alarming rate and have placed natural life systems at risk. The climate crisis has the potential to compromise any positive progress there has been in global health thus far.

Planetary health is the health of human civilisation and the natural systems on which it depends. It highlights that human and natural systems are intrinsically interrelated.

Currently, only 15% of medical schools include climate change as part of their teaching, and this chapter explains why there needs to be a drive to increase the amount of time and resources put into teaching medical students and healthcare professionals about the climate crisis [1].

The chapter will explore the reciprocal relationship between the healthcare sector's role in contributing to the climate crisis and the impacts that the climate crisis has on healthcare. It will then go on to discuss some of the ways in which we can combat the climate crisis and look at some ideas for sustainability.

U. Rai
London, UK

N. Olsen (✉)
School of Medicine, Cardiff University, Cardiff, UK
e-mail: natalie@olsenhome.co.uk

A. Fiander, G. Fry (eds.), *A Healthcare Students Introduction to Global Health*, https://doi.org/10.1007/978-3-031-66563-9_24

24.1 How Does the Provision of Healthcare Contribute to the Global Climate Crisis?

24.1.1 Global Healthcare Contributions

In 2017, the World Bank, along with Health Care Without Harm, estimated that globally the healthcare sector generated and emitted 2.6 billion out of 52 billion tonnes of carbon dioxide in 2011, which was about 5% of all global carbon dioxide emissions [2].

The healthcare sector in 36 countries of the Organisation for Economic Cooperation and Development Organisation (OECD), India and China were responsible for 4.4% of the total carbon dioxide emissions from these countries [3].

If healthcare were to be considered a country, it would be the fifth largest contributor in the world. This would place it above Japan and Brazil [2].

Antibiotic presence has been traced in 65% of 711 rivers worldwide [4]. This can have serious impacts in terms of antibiotics being biologically active molecules that have effects on humans as well as contributing to antibiotic resistance.

- In the Danube, seven different types of antibiotics were detected.
- In Bangladesh, concentrations of metronidazole in a river were 300 times higher than the limit deemed 'safe' for the environment [4].

24.1.2 Medical Plastic Waste

- There are huge issues around single use plastic in hospitals around the world, since 2% of all global plastic is medical waste.
- Twenty-five per cent of waste generated by a hospital is plastic. It was found that a single hysterectomy procedure can produce up to 20 pounds of waste, most of which is plastic.
- The WHO reported that 85% of hospital waste is non-infectious, and most waste is recyclable. Most medical waste currently finds itself in landfilled or it incinerated.

24.1.3 Global Healthcare Footprint by Categories

The overall carbon footprint has been broken down using the Greenhouse Gas Protocol (GHG) emission scopes. The GHG is used by the UK government as an independent standard to follow when reporting greenhouse gas emissions. NHS Wales's procurement carbon footprint for 2018–19 broke down the overall carbon footprint by the GHG emission scopes [5].

1. Scope 1—direct emissions generated directly by the combustion of gas and other fuels from healthcare facilities.

   • 13%

2. Scope 2—indirect emissions generated by purchased electricity, steam, cooling and heating.

   • 6%

3. Scope 3—emissions generated from the healthcare supply chain, the production, transportation, use and disposal of products.

   • 81%

As healthcare professionals, it is important to recognise that we can make a difference on an individual level by addressing scopes 1 and 2. Even the smallest changes such as remembering to turn off lights in corridors or in rooms that are not being used will reduce indirect emissions, and anaesthetists can challenge their use of damaging gases to cut down direct emissions.

Emissions of scope 3 can be further subdivided into upstream and downstream activities. Scope 3 can be reduced by the NHS and make a huge difference in both upstream and downstream activities.

'Upstream activities' include product supply, transport and assets of the operation of the organisation.

'Downstream activities' refer to product outputs and assets excluding operational ownership.

24.1.4 NHS Wales Procurement Carbon Footprint

The NHS Wales's procurement carbon footprint for 2018–19 was reported to be around 1 million tonnes of carbon dioxide, with an estimated cost of £1965m of direct Wales spend [5]. Procurement accounts for 62% emissions, with drugs and pharmaceuticals contributing 35% of all procurement emissions [5].

24.1.5 Anaesthetic Gases as Greenhouse Gases

The gases used for anaesthesia are greenhouse gases and include hydrofluorocarbons such as sevoflurane, isoflurane and desflurane and nitrous oxide. After these gases have been used, they are expelled into the atmosphere and contribute to the climate crisis.

Almost 4 million metric tonnes of healthcare emissions come from the use of anaesthetic gases and metered dose inhalers. They contribute around 0.6% of all healthcare's global climate impact and 5% of the NHS's carbon footprint [6].

Anaesthetists should be aware of the contributions the drugs they use have on the climate crisis and review whether they need to use specific gases, or if there are alternative, more sustainable ways for anaesthesia.

Many anaesthetists have their own personal preferential gases, and this is influenced by the patient, surgical and anaesthetic factors. Anaesthetic gases are commonly excluded when suggesting ways for the healthcare sector to become more sustainable as they are considered a medical necessity and play a key role in treatment and care. It is therefore important that anaesthetists challenge the use of each gas daily.

Desflurane is the most damaging anaesthetic gas, and the Montreal Protocol is planning to move away from chlorofluorocarbon use. One hour's use of desflurane equates to 230 miles travelled by car [7].

24.1.6 NHS Is a Large Public Sector Contributor to the UK's Greenhouse Gas Emissions

- Every year, NHS England produces more carbon dioxide than all passenger planes taking off from Heathrow.
- The NHS produces 5.4% of the UK's greenhouse gas emissions.
- Over 1 million tonnes of carbon dioxide were emitted by NHS Wales in 2018–19. This has an estimated cost of £1965 million.
- Sixty-five per cent of NHS's carbon footprint is due to procurement, including pharmaceutical and medical devices.

24.2 How Can We Make Healthcare More Sustainable?

24.2.1 Sustainability

In the broadest sense, sustainability refers to the ability to maintain or support a process continuously over time and seeks to prevent the depletion of natural or physical resources. It focuses on meeting the needs of the present without compromising the ability of future generations to meet their needs. If we continue our current medical practice, there will be insufficient resources to meet the needs of our future patients' [8]. Hence, the need for sustainable healthcare is crucial.

To achieve sustainable healthcare, there are a range of key players which need to be considered. This is summarised in Fig. 24.1.

Fig. 24.1 Different stakeholders involved in sustainable healthcare

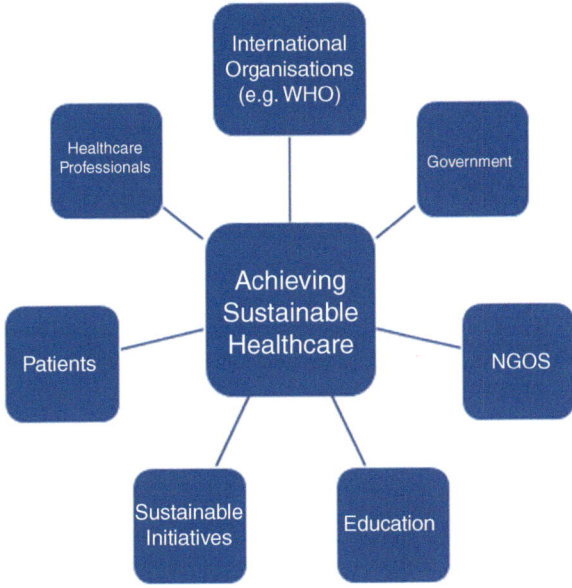

24.2.2 *Patients*

Increasing patient awareness is a key factor since they are the consumer of healthcare services [9]. If patients were aware of their ecological footprint, they may behave in a more eco-conscious way. Here are a few examples [10]:

- If a patient does not finish their entire course of tablets, they may return the rest to the pharmacist. This way, the tablets can be disposed correctly, and this is a better alternative than simply throwing them out.
- The means of transport that a patient takes could be influenced. They may opt to take the bus instead of taking a car, which reduces carbon dioxide emissions. In addition, some may even decide to walk or use a bike—becoming more active!
- Patients will be more likely to attend appointments. A study conducted by Family Medicine highlighted that 41% of participants did not understand the impact of not showing up to their appointment. Therefore, it is key that patients need to be aware of the effects. For example, every GP appointment missed costs the NHS £35.

24.2.3 Healthcare Initiatives—Recycling

Single use medical supplies are a huge problem for the environment creating massive plastic waste. This issue becomes greater with pandemics, such as COVID-19, where there is a requirement to wear disposal face masks. Recycling can be a solution to this problem. Recycling can:

- Prevent the waste being incinerated and therefore reduce the carbon dioxide emissions that are produced which speed up the greenhouse effect. According to the WHO, as much as 90% of all medical waste is incinerated [11].
- Reduce leakage of harmful or toxic waste into the surrounding environment.
- Reduce the need for raw materials, such as oil, to create single use plastic items. This will prevent environmental degradation, oil spillages and increase biodiversity in areas around the world.

To implement widespread recycling, it is important to challenge the ideas around recycling. There is a belief that infectious diseases could be spread with recycled equipment and hence would-be hesitancy in using the equipment. However, only 15% of healthcare waste is classed as 'hazardous' and therefore the potential of recycling could be fruitful [12].

24.2.4 Healthcare Professionals

It is important that healthcare professionals operate in a sustainable fashion. Applying eco-friendly protocols to simple procedures could be beneficial environmentally and economically. Some examples include:

- The way healthcare professionals communicate is still heavily dominated with paper within the NHS. Matt Hancock, when Health and Social Care Secretary, pushed for a modern version of the NHS using a secure email provider [13]. In December 2018, Hancock announced a fax machine ban within the NHS so that these can no longer be bought. At the time NHS hospital trusts owned over 8000 fax machines.
- There are benefits to using emails including greater security, faster communication and less environmental impact. A letter lost in the post can have a significant medical effect.
- Doctors and other health professionals frequently travel around the globe for conferences and research. The adoption of video conferencing software, such as Zoom, could be a better alternative. Conferences can be recorded; more people can attend due to the easier accessibility, and it reduces greenhouse emissions.

24.2.5 *International Organisations*

There are a range of international organisations that aim to shape healthcare around the world to make it more sustainable.

- Health Care Without Harm (HCWH) is a non-profit network of hospitals, healthcare systems and local authorities throughout Europe whose aim is to transform healthcare by reducing its ecological footprint. They have had success in phasing out mercury based-medical devices, which bioaccumulate in the environment and negatively impact human and environmental health. They replaced mercury with cheaper and safer equipment and were able to change global practice. There are numerous examples which can be explored on their website [14].
- The United Nations have also encouraged sustainable healthcare practices through their Sustainable Development Goals (SDGs). Introduced in 2015, many of these can be applicable to healthcare services. For example, responsible consumption and production, good health and wellbeing and climate change. These goals were integrated into HCWH policies and how they approached projects.

References

1. Greenwald L, Blanchard O, Hayden C, Sheffield P. Climate and health education: A critical review at one medical school. Front Public Health. 2022;10:1092359.
2. Health Care Without Harm (HCWH). Health care's climate footprint 2019 [10/11/2020]. Available from: https://www.arup.com/perspectives/publications/research/section/healthcares-climate-footprint
3. World Health Organisation. COP26 key messages on climate change 2020 [10/11/2020]. Available from: https://www.who.int/publications/i/item/cop26-key-messages-on-climate-change-and-health
4. National Geographic. First global look finds most rivers awash with antibiotics 2019 [11/11/2020]. Available from: https://www.nationalgeographic.com/environment/2019/05/hundreds-of-worlds-rivers-contain-dangerous-levels-antibiotics/
5. NHS Wales Carbon Footprint. Scope 1, 2 & 3 Carbon Footprint Assessment for NHS Wales 2019 [10/11/2020]. Available from: https://gov.wales/sites/default/files/publications/2020-09/nhswales-carbon-footprint-2018-19.pdf
6. Whiting A, Tennison I, Roschnik S, Collins M. Surgery and the NHS carbon footprint. Bull Royal Coll Surg Engl. 2020;102(5):182–5.
7. Secretariat UEPO. Environmental effects of stratospheric Ozone depletion, UV radiation, and interactions with climate change 2023. Available from: https://ozone.unep.org/system/files/documents/EEAP-2022-Assessment-Report-May2023.pdf
8. Mollenkamp DT. What is sustainability? 2023. Available from: https://www.investopedia.com/terms/s/sustainability.asp
9. Lacy NL, Paulman A, Reuter MD, Lovejoy B. Why we don't come: patient perceptions on no-shows. Ann Fam Med. 2004;2(6):541–5.
10. Zafar S. This is how we can make healthcare more sustainable 2023. Available from: https://www.cleantechloops.com/healthcare-sustainable/
11. Ngo H. How do you fix healthcare's medical waste problem?. 2020.

12. Linnenkoper K. Medical waste may be difficult to recyle, but is hardly a bio-hazard 2018. Available from: https://recyclinginternational.com/latest-articles/editors-top-picks/medical-waste-may-be-difficult-to-recycle-but-is-hardly-a-bio-hazard/16883/
13. Department of Health and Social Care. Matt Hancock: email must replace paper in NHS. 2019.
14. Health Care Without Harm (HCWH). Mercury in health care 2019. Available from: https://noharm-global.org/issues/global/mercury-health-care

Chapter 25
'Is Planetary Health More Important than Individual Health'

Neve James and Hannah Cox

25.1 What Is Planetary Health?

Planetary health describes how the health and well-being of the planet are interconnected. We rely on the planet for food, water, oxygen as well as other resources that are essential for our survival. However, as a direct result of our actions, the supply of these resources is threatened. Disruption to the earth's natural ecosystems is impacting the availability and quality of these resources, which in turn threatens the long-term survival of the human population. One of the principal pillars of the NHS is to do no harm. While this is usually referring to the treatment of patients, it can also be applied in the context of sustainable healthcare. If treating patients today impacts the environment to an extent that it is compromising the earth for future generations, then this is not sustainable. Henceforth, harm is being done, and the oath isn't being upheld.

25.1.1 Healthcare's Role in Climate Change

The NHS plays a huge role in climate change and contributes 4% [1] of the UK's greenhouse gas emissions. Most emissions are produced by healthcare supply chains, in particular the production of 'pharmaceuticals, chemicals and medical equipment' [2]. Worldwide healthcare systems produce 4% of global CO_2 emissions [3]. As a large contributor to greenhouse emissions, the NHS can play an instrumental role in meeting targets. Therefore, in 2008, a sustainable development unit was created to assess the carbon footprint of the NHS and work to reduce it.

N. James (✉) · H. Cox (✉)
School of Medicine, Cardiff University, Cardiff, UK
e-mail: coxhm@cardiff.ac.uk

25.1.2   The Link Between Health and Climate Change

Increasing global temperatures in combination with more extreme weather conditions can directly lead to injuries, illness and deaths. It can also alter breeding grounds for diseases resulting in an increase in many diseases such as malaria and dengue fever, while rising sea levels are expected to increase water-borne viruses such as cholera. Healthcare services may be ill-prepared for these changes, with 80% of communicable and non-communicable diseases being influenced by environmental factors.

Climate change will have a large impact on food chains and water supplies. Our food production is dependent on the climate to produce the right environment for crops to grow. Therefore, a change in the climate may result in a reduction in crop growth in areas, leading to food shortages and malnutrition. Rising sea levels could lead to many people being displaced into areas that don't have adequate healthcare services [4].

Climate change will ultimately affect all populations; however, factors such as geographical location, climate, age and health infrastructure are all variables that result in some populations being disproportionately affected [5]. Children from lower socioeconomic countries are more vulnerable and will be exposed for longer, while the elderly and those with underlying health conditions are expected to be impacted more severely. Costal populations are also understandably at risk and may not have the infrastructure to manage rising sea levels.

25.1.3   What Is More Important, the Health of the Individual or the Health of the Planet?

25.2   Individual Health

Why might healthcare systems prioritise the health of the individual over that of the planet? Working in healthcare is about striking a balance between best meeting the needs of the patient and protecting the planet from harm by practising in a sustainable way.

Take Entonox as an example, an effective, safe and cheap drug that is routinely used as analgesia for women in labour. Entonox contains nitrous oxide which is almost 300 times more potent as a greenhouse gas than carbon dioxide [6]. This poses a medical dilemma for healthcare professionals. One study indicated that most pregnant women receiving Entonox gas had less labour pain (91.8%) and were satisfied with it (98%) [7]. It is also a non-invasive means of pain relief. However, do its beneficial analgesic effects for labouring women justify its adverse effects on the planet?

In 2021, Newcastle Hospitals implemented machines designed to collect and destroy nitrous oxide from exhaled gas and air. These Mobile Destruction Units provide a potential solution to the above conundrum by balancing patient care and the health of the planet [6].

Without alternative medications with a lower carbon footprint, doctors find themselves in a challenging position. The development and clinical trial process involved in licensing a new and sustainable drug is lengthy. Therefore, doctors are compelled to choose the best possible treatment option for the patient which may not necessarily be the most sustainable one.

Implementing sustainable changes within the healthcare system is expensive and would require a diversion of funding to create systems and equipment that are both fit for purpose and environment friendly. This is especially difficult in healthcare systems that are already stretched financially. In addition, hospital staff simply do not have the time or energy to generate and implement new sustainable ideas alongside providing patient care.

25.3 Planetary Health

Environmentalism warns us of the impending threat that increased planetary neglect poses to human health. In the Lancet's 2019 report on climate change, it was found that rising temperatures and worsening heat waves are increasing the risk of cardiovascular, kidney, respiratory and cerebrovascular disease, as well as heatstroke. This phenomenon occurs as rapid rises in temperature compromise the body's ability to regulate temperature which increases an individual's risk of developing the aforementioned illnesses [8].

Flooding, made worse by rising sea levels, contributes to death and injury. Flooding also contaminates drinking water, therefore playing a role in the spread of infectious disease, alongside hotter temperatures. Those affected by these harsh conditions are unsurprisingly at an increased risk of mental health problems [9]. Furthermore, a discussion about climate change is incomplete without covering air pollution. To date, air pollution has contributed towards roughly seven million deaths globally [8]. The Lancet's findings also show that poor air quality damages all vital organs, with effects accumulating over time [8].

All these points evidence the link between the planet's health and our own. In doing so, it illuminates a crucial fact—focusing on planetary health is as important, if not more important, than simply treating individual health problems. By tackling the environmental factors that impact a range of health concerns, the need to treat individuals presenting with such issues can be reduced. As the link between planetary health and individual health is so clear, the healthcare sector is bound to an ethical and professional obligation to incorporate environmentally sustainable practices. As per the Hippocratic Oath *do no harm*, it would be contradictory for the healthcare sector to contribute to environmental harm when this will lead to more health issues in humans and increased demand for, and pressure on, the healthcare sector.

Climate change, like smoking, is a silent killer. While its effects are disproportionately seen in lower-income countries, higher-income countries (which ironically produce significantly more greenhouse gases) will remain relatively unaffected until it is too late to act [10]. The disproportionate impact of climate change on vulnerable populations means that its repercussions on health are also not felt equally [11]. For instance, climate change will displace susceptible populations and thus change the geographical distribution of infectious disease [11].

In higher resource countries, the biggest challenge will not be heat shock or malaria, but rather the arrival of people from parts of the world made uninhabitable by the cumulative effects of climate change [10]. Although the effects are yet to be seen, this displacement of large populations has the potential to introduce disease, increase food scarcity and place strain on healthcare systems. This illustrates how the effects of climate change will silently creep up on higher-income countries, only really being felt once the damage is irreversible.

Collectively acting, by reducing fossil fuel emissions, can drastically improve health outcomes. For example, walking or cycling instead of driving can yield physical and mental health benefits [10]. Moreover, shifting towards more plant-based diets can decrease carbon emissions and is beneficial to our own personal health [10].

Taking all of this into consideration, some would argue that planetary health measures take precedence over individual health. Sustainable practices have the potential to be more holistic and address health issues on a worldwide scale for the long-term.

25.3.1   Case Study Example: What can be Done from a Health Perspective in the United Kingdom?

The National Health Service

- Switching to treatments that have a lower carbon footprint, while not compromising the care of the patient.
- As mentioned previously, 16% of the NHS footprint is due to travel of both patients and staff, which is where telemedicine could play a large role in the future of medicine. While it cannot replace face-to-face consultations, it would reduce any unnecessary travel for patients that can be seen and managed remotely.
- A reduction in air pollution from travel will also help those with respiratory conditions, as the pollution can trigger and exacerbate their symptoms.
- Shifting care from treatment to prevention would also have better outcomes for the patient and a reduced impact on the planet.

- Increased prudence when prescribing medications, particularly for some mental health conditions and loneliness which may be better treated with social prescribing.

    Individuals

- Incentivising walking or cycling to reduce carbon output from vehicle travel. This would also promote time outside and physical exercise to benefit both mental and physical health—whilst not contributing to climate change.
- Switching from meat based to more plant-based diets reduces cholesterol absorption and synthesis, hence decreasing the need for statins as well as having a lower carbon footprint and water usage.

References

1. Naylor C. What if the NHS were to go carbon neutral? The King's Fund. 2021. https://www.kingsfund.org.uk/reports/thenhsif/what-if-carbon-neutral-nhs/%20. Accessed 21 Apr 2021.
2. Tennison I, et al. Health care's response to climate change: a carbon footprint assessment of the NHS in England. Lancet Planet Health. 2021;5(2):e84–92.
3. Pichler P, Jaccard I, Weisz U, Weisz H. 2019. International comparison of health care carbon footprints.
4. CDC. 2021. Climate effects on health. https://www.cdc.gov/climateandhealth/effects/ Accessed 21 Apr 2021.
5. WHO. 2018. Climate and health. https://www.who.int/news-room/fact-sheets/detail/climate-change-and-health. Accessed 21 Apr 2021
6. Newcastle Hospitals NHS Foundation Trust. 2021. Newcastle Hospitals become first in the UK to use climate-friendly gas and air during labour. https://www.newcastle-hospitals.nhs.uk/news/newcastle-hospitals-become-first-in-the-uk-to-use-climate-friendly-gas-and-air-during-labour/. Accessed: 20 Apr 2021.
7. Pasha H, Basirat Z, Hajahmadi M, Bakhtiari A, Faramarzi M, Salmalian H. Maternal expectations and experiences of labor analgesia with nitrous oxide. Iran Red Crescent Med J. 2012.
8. Watts N, et al. The 2019 report of The Lancet Countdown on health and climate change: ensuring that the health of a child born today is not defined by a changing climate. Lancet. 2019;394(10211):1836–78.
9. Health Declares. Climate change and health. 2021. https://healthdeclares.org/the-science/climate-change-and-health/. Accessed 24 Apr 2021.
10. Thompson T, Ballard T. Sustainable medicine: good for the environment, good for people. Br J General Pract. 2011;61(582):3–4.
11. Climate Just. 2021. Who is vulnerable? https://www.climatejust.org.uk/who-vulnerable. Accessed 24 Apr 2021.